Level 2

BTEC
SPORT
ASSESSMENT GUIDE

CW00954189

Unit 1 FITNESS FOR SPORT AND EXERCISE

Unit 2 PRACTICAL SPORTS PERFORMANCE

JENNIFER STAFFORD-BROWN
SIMON REA, KATHERINE HOWARD
AND ANDREW BARDSLEY

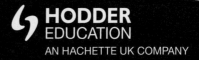

HODDER
EDUCATION
AN HACHETTE UK COMPANY

The sample learner answers provided in this assessment guide are intended to give guidance on how a learner might approach generating evidence for each assessment criterion. Answers do not necessarily include all of the evidence required to meet each assessment criterion. Assessor comments intend to highlight how sample answers might be improved to help learners meet the requirements of the grading criterion but are provided as a guide only. Sample answers and assessor guidance have not been verified by Edexcel and any information provided in this guide should not replace your own internal verification process.

Any work submitted as evidence for assessment for this unit must be the learner's own. Submitting as evidence, in whole or in part, any material taken from this guide will be regarded as plagiarism. Hodder Education accepts no responsibility for learners plagiarising work from this guide that does or does not meet the assessment criteria.

The sample assignment briefs are provided as a guide to how you might assess the evidence required for all or part of the internal assessment of this Unit. They have not been verified or endorsed by Edexcel and should be internally verified through your own Lead Internal Verifier as with any other assignment briefs, and/or checked through the BTEC assignment checking service.

Orders: please contact Bookpoint Ltd, 130 Milton Park, Abingdon, Oxon OX14 4SB. Telephone: (44) 01235 827720. Fax: (44) 01235 400454. Lines are open from 9.00–5.00, Monday to Saturday, with a 24-hour message answering service. You can also order through our website www.hoddereducation.co.uk

If you have any comments to make about this, or any of our other titles, please send them to educationenquiries@hodder.co.uk

British Library Cataloguing in Publication Data

A catalogue record for this title is available from the British Library

ISBN: 978 1 444 1 86628

Published 2013

Impression number   10 9 8 7 6 5 4 3 2 1

Year   2016 2015 2014 2013

Copyright © 2013 Jennifer Stafford-Brown, Simon Rea, Katherine Howard and Andrew Bardsley

Cover photo © Stockbyte/Photolibrary Group Ltd/Getty Images

Typeset by Integra Software Services Pvt, Ltd., Pondicherry, India

Printed in Dubai for Hodder Education,
an Hachette UK Company,
338 Euston Road,
London NW1 3BH

Contents

A note on the authors

This book consists of two units;
Unit 1 Fitness for Sport and Exercise was written by Katherine Howard and Andrew Bardsley.
Unit 2 Practical Sports Performance was written by Jennifer Stafford-Brown and Simon Rea.

For attention of the learner

You are not allowed to copy any information from this book and use it as your own evidence. That would count as plagiarism, which is taken very seriously and may result in disqualification. If you are in any doubt at all please speak to your teacher.

Command words

You will find the following command words in the external assessment and assessment criteria for each unit.

Analyse	Identify the factors that apply and state how these are related. Explain the importance of each one.
Apply/use	Put skills/knowledge/understanding into action in a particular context, or use it to achieve a specific goal or target.
Compare and contrast	Identify the main factors relating to two or more items/situations, and explain the similarities and differences, and in some cases say which is best and why.
Describe	Give a clear description that includes all the relevant features – think of it as 'painting a picture with words'.
Explain	Provide details and give reasons and/or evidence to support the arguments being made. Start by introducing the topic then give the 'how' or 'why'.
Produce	Create a specific document or plan.
Review	Examine a topic or an item to make sure that it is correct or to provide a report on the quality of a document/report/item.

Unit 1
Fitness for Sport and Exercise

Unit 1, Fitness for Sport and Exercise, is an externally assessed, compulsory unit with three learning aims:

- Learning aim A: Know about the components of fitness and the principles of training
- Learning aim B: Explore different fitness training methods
- Learning aim C: Investigate fitness testing to determine fitness levels.

Unit 1 is a core unit and its content underpins the other BTEC sport units. Learning aim A looks at the components of physical and skill-related fitness and principles of training. Learning aim B covers the various training methods that can be used to develop the different components of fitness and learning aim C focuses on fitness tests.

The unit is divided in to two sections. The first section contains the content of the learning aim, broken down in to bite-sized chunks. Each topic is covered and you can tick them off as you study them.

The second section contains two sample external assessments. You will be given 1 hour to complete the external assessment for this unit and the marks are out of 50. Your assessment will take place by an online, computer-based test and our two sample external assessments are designed to show you the types of questions, and question formats, you might face. Answers for the two sample external assessments can be found at the end of the book.

Learning aim A
Know about the components of fitness and the principles of training

Topic A.1 Components of physical fitness

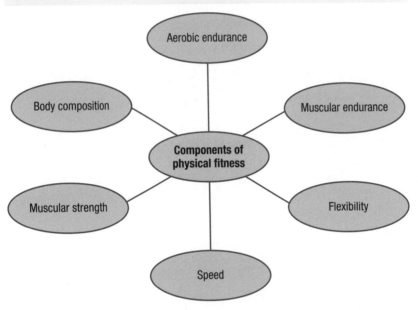

You will need to know the definition of each of the six different components of fitness.

Aerobic endurance

Aerobic endurance is the ability of the cardiorespiratory system to work efficiently, supplying nutrients and oxygen to working muscles during sustained physical activity.

There are alternative names for this component of physical fitness; these are:

- cardiorespiratory fitness
- cardiorespiratory endurance, or
- aerobic fitness.

Remember that the cardiorespiratory system consists of the cardiovascular system, which includes the heart, blood

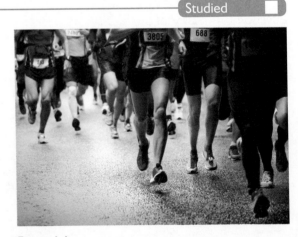

Figure 1.1

and blood vessels; and the respiratory system, which includes the lungs and airways.

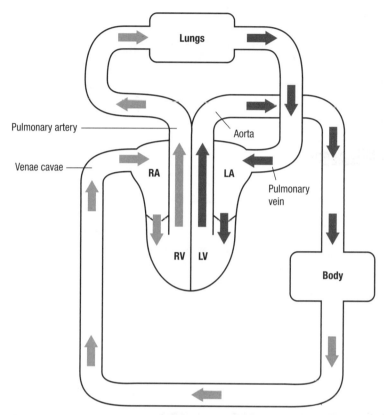

Figure 1.2 The cardiorespiratory system

The cardiorespiratory system is responsible for taking in and using oxygen from the air that is breathed in and also for transporting nutrients and oxygen around the body. It also removes waste products such as carbon dioxide and lactic acid.

Muscular endurance

Studied

This is the ability of the muscular system to work efficiently. A person with muscular endurance is able to have their muscles continue contracting over a period of time against a light to moderate fixed resistance load.

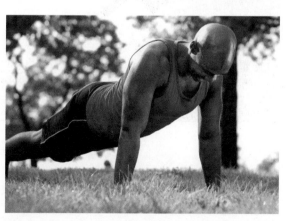

Figure 1.3

3

Flexibility

This means having an adequate range of motion in all joints of the body so that you are able to carry out all of the movements that are required every day. It also means the ability to move a joint fluidly through its complete range of movement.

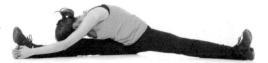

Figure 1.4

Speed

This is the distance a person travels divided by the time taken to travel that distance. Speed is measured in metres per second (m/s). The faster an athlete is able to run over a set distance, the greater their speed.

There are three main types of speed:

- Accelerative speed – these are sprints up to 30 metres.
- Pure speed – these are sprints up to 60 meters.
- Speed endurance – these are sprints with a short recovery period in between.

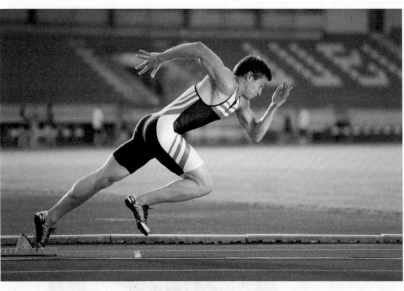

Figure 1.5

Accelerative speed

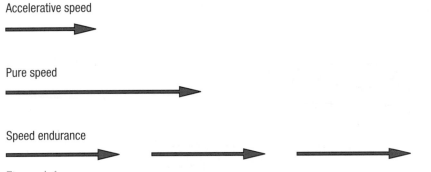

Pure speed

Speed endurance

Figure 1.6

Muscular strength

Studied ☐

This is the maximum force (in kg or N) that can be generated by a muscle or muscle group.

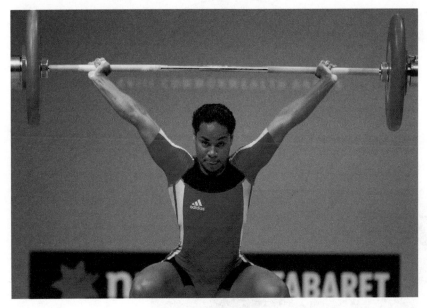

Figure 1.7

Body composition

Studied ☐

This is the relative ratio of fat mass to fat-free mass (vital organs, muscle, bone) in the body.

Topic A.2 Components of skill-related fitness

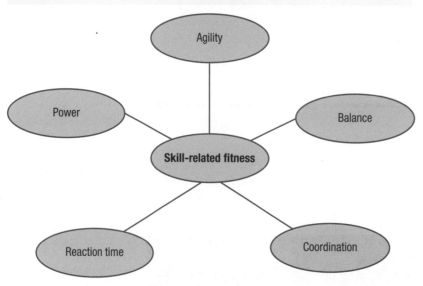

Agility

Studied ☐

This is the ability of a sports performer to quickly and precisely move or change direction without losing balance or time.

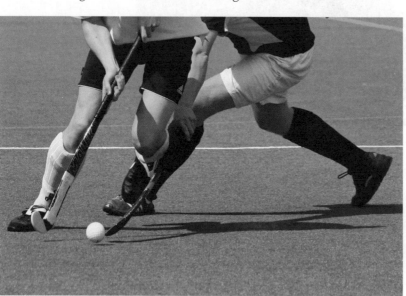

Figure 1.8

Balance

Studied ☐

This is the ability to maintain centre of mass over a base of support.

There are two types of balance:

- static balance
- dynamic balance.

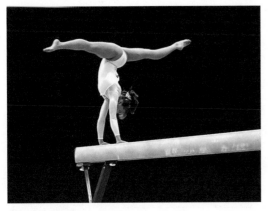

Figure 1.9

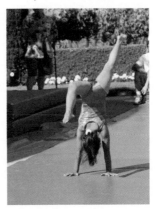

Figure 1.10

Coordination

Studied ☐

This is the smooth flow of movement needed to perform a motor task efficiently and accurately.

Power

Studied ☐

This is the product of strength and speed and is expressed as the work done in a unit of time.

An example of power can be seen when we throw an object or perform a sprint start.

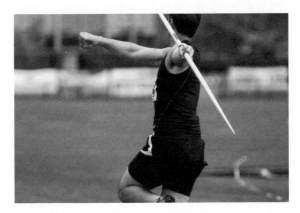

Figure 1.11

Reaction time

Studied ☐

This is time the taken for a sports performer to respond to a stimulus and the initiation of their response.

Learning aim A: Know about the components of fitness and the principles of training

7

Topic A.3 Why fitness components are important for successful participation in given sports

Meeting physical demands to reach optimal performance

Studied ☐

Having high levels of each of the required fitness components for a specific sport is very important in order for the sports performer to successfully meet the physical demands of the sport and reach their highest levels of performance.

Meeting skill-related demands to reach optimal performance

Studied ☐

Some sports rely on high levels of skill and, in these cases, having high levels of each of the required skill-related components for the sport is essential in order for the sports person to perform successfully.

Performing efficiently

Studied ☐

Efficient performance is also important so that energy is not wasted.

Giving consideration to the type of event/position played

Studied ☐

In some sports, different members of a team may require different types of physical fitness and skill-related fitness. For example, a goal keeper in football will require high levels of power, speed and strength, fast reaction times and good coordination in order to perform their role well, whereas a striker would need high levels of muscular endurance, aerobic endurance, speed, power and agility to perform well in their position.

Topic A.4 Exercise intensity and how it can be determined

Intensity

Studied ☐

For your external assessment you will need to be able to measure heart rate (HR) and apply HR intensity to fitness training methods.

Intensity is how hard an individual trains. Individuals should train at different training intensities depending on the fitness results that they want to attain.

Target zones and training thresholds

Studied ☐

The different training levels are called **training zones** and these can be used to work out **target zones** and **training thresholds**.

A target zone is the range of heart rate values an individual should work within in order for training intensity to be effective.

Training thresholds are the minimum heart rate values a person has to exercise at in order to improve aerobic or anaerobic fitness.

Calculating HR max

Studied ☐

In order to calculate training zones, you first of all need to work out the maximum heart rate (HR max) for an individual. This is measured in beats per minute (bpm).

HR max = 220 minus age (in years)

So for a 16 year old:

HR max = 220 – 16 = 204 beats per minute (bpm)

Calculating the recommended training zone

Studied ☐

The recommended training zone for cardiovascular health and fitness is 60–85% HR max.

You will need to be able to calculate 60–85% HR max for people of different ages.

To work out the training zone at 60–85% of maximal heart rate for an 18 year old:

HR Max = 220 – 18 = 202 bpm

Training range is:

60%: HR Max x 60/100

202 x 60/100 = 121 bpm

85%: HR Max x 80/100

202 x 85/100 = 172 bpm

Therefore, the training zone for an 18 year old is 121 to 172 beats per minute. This means the individual should make sure their heart rate is between these numbers in order to ensure that they are training at the correct intensity.

Always round up or down to a whole number – bpm is always measured in whole numbers.

Always include the units in your answer if you have the option – this may give you extra marks!

The Borg Rating of Perceived Exertion (RPE) Scale

The RPE Scale can be used as a measure of exercise intensity. The scale ranges from 6 (rest) to 20 (exhaustion).

Rating of perceived exertion (RPE)	
6	No exertion at all
7	Extremely light
8	
9	Very light
10	Light
11	Somewhat hard
12	
13	
14	
15	Hard
16	
17	Very hard
18	
19	Extremely hard
20	Maximum exertion

Table 1.1

RPE and heart rate

The number stated on the scale can be multiplied by 10 to get an estimate of heart rate during the workout.

RPE x 10 = HR (bpm)

If an individual was working at level 15 on the RPE scale, their HR could be worked out:

15 x 10 = 150 bpm

Topic A.5 The basic principles of training (FITT)

FITT is an acronym for the different principles of training that should be used when designing personal training programmes.

Frequency

The number of training sessions completed over a period of time, usually per week.

Intensity

How hard an individual will train; this is usually expressed as a percentage of maximum intensity.

Time

How long an individual will train for each session.

Type

How an individual will train by selecting a training method to improve a specific component of fitness and/or their sports performance.

When applying the FITT principles in a training programme, you are basically asking the following questions:

- How often?
- How hard?
- How long?
- What do you do?

For your external assessment, you will need to be able to apply the FITT principles to training methods, regimes and given exercise situations.

Topic A.6 Additional principles of training

Progressive overload

Overload is where an athlete keeps working harder than they used to in order to ensure that they continue to gain fitness. This continued increase in intensity (how hard they work) is called progressive overload. In order to progress, training needs to be demanding enough to cause the body to adapt in order to improve performance.

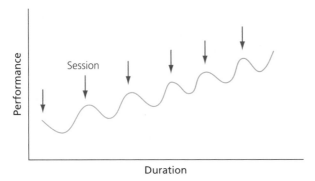

Figure 1.12 Progressive overload

Specificity

This means that any fitness gain will be specific to the muscles or systems to which the training is applied. As different types of training will produce different results, it is important to make sure that training is specific to the sport that an individual is competing in. For example, if you are training for a marathon, you would need to have lots of distance running in your training programme – you would not improve your running performance if your training only included swimming!

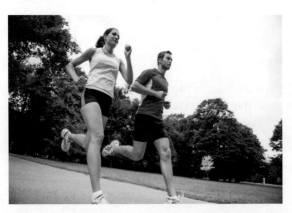

Figure 1.13

Individual differences/needs

Studied ☐

The programme should be designed to meet personal training goals and needs. These are determined from the personal goals and competition schedule of the individual.

The programme should also include different exercises, activities and timings to prevent the individual from becoming bored with the training programme.

Adaptation

Studied ☐

This is where the body changes to cope with the extra loads and stresses applied to the body systems during training.

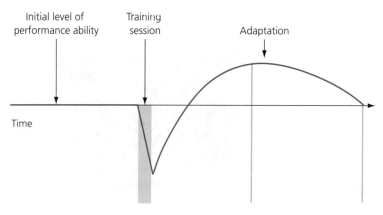

Adaptation after a training session.

Figure 1.14 Adaptation

Adaptation occurs during the recovery period after the training session is completed.

Reversibility

Studied ☐

If training stops, or if the intensity of training is not sufficient to cause adaptation, then the training effects are reversed and the body will return to its previous fitness level. This is sometimes referred to as the 'use it or lose it' principle.

Variation

Studied ☐

It is important to include variety in the training regime otherwise the individual may become bored, which makes it difficult to maintain enjoyment and motivation to train.

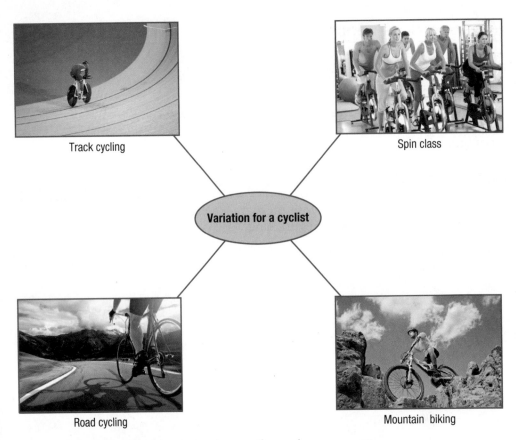

Track cycling

Spin class

Variation for a cyclist

Road cycling

Mountain biking

Notice that each type of training is specific to the competition sport, so the training is still specific! The occasional exercise that is not specific to the sport can also be included in a training programme for variation, which helps to improve some components of physical fitness, such as yoga for flexibility training or swimming to help with aerobic endurance.

Rest and recovery

Most athletes will have at least one rest day a week to give their body time to adapt to the training that they have completed.

Application of training principles

For the external assessment, you will need to be able to apply the principles of training to different training methods, different training regimes and different exercise settings.

Examples of some of these are shown below.

An example of a fitness exercise session to improve aerobic fitness and muscular endurance fitness:

Type of training	Description of amount	Guidance
CV training – warm-up	3–5 minutes.	This involves a gradual increase of intensity to raise the heart rate steadily.
Flexibility	2–3 dynamic stretches.	These stretches involve moving the joints and muscles through the full range of movement in a controlled manner to replicate movements coming up in the main session.
Resistance 1	4–5 exercises to cover the main muscle groups (pecs, lats, glutes, quads and hamstrings).	High reps and low weights to improve muscular endurance. Exercises could include free weights, resistance machines or cable exercises.
CV training	Between 5 and 20 minutes dependent upon the goals of the individual.	Could involve steady state work or intervals. For aerobic endurance, this could involve running, rowing or cycling.
Resistance 2	4–5 exercises to cover a selection of the minor muscle groups (biceps, triceps, deltoids, calves).	High reps and low weights to improve muscular endurance. Exercises could include free weights, resistance machines or cable exercises.
CV training	Between 5 and 20 minutes dependent upon the goals of the individual.	Could involve steady state work or intervals. For aerobic endurance, this could involve running, rowing or cycling.
Core training	2–3 exercises to cover the abdominals, back muscles (erector spinae) and obliques.	This could include dynamic exercises, such as sit-ups, crunches or back extensions or static exercises, such as the plank or a bridge.
CV training – cool-down	3–5 minutes.	This involves a gradual decrease of intensity to lower the heart rate steadily.
Flexibility	8–10 stretches on all the muscles worked in the session.	This would include developmental stretches on those muscles which are tight (e.g. pecs, hamstrings) and static stretches on all the other muscles worked.

Table 1.2

A typical training session for an untrained beginner may look like this:

Type of training	Name of exercise	Amount
CV training – warm-up	Treadmill	5 minutes.
Flexibility	Dynamic stretches: chest, back, legs	x 10 on each exercise.
Resistance 1	Squats Bench press Seated row Leg extension Leg flexion	2 x 15 on each exercise with 20–30 seconds rest between sets and exercises.
CV training	Rower	5–10 minutes.
Resistance 2	Shoulder press Bicep curls Tricep press Calf raises	2 x 15 on each exercise with 20–30 seconds rest between sets and exercises.
CV training	Static bike	3–5 minutes.
Core training	Sit-ups on stability ball Back extensions on stability ball	2 x 10 repetitions on each exercise.
CV training – cool-down	Treadmill	3–5 minutes.
Flexibility	Quads Hamstrings (developmental) Pecs (developmental) Lats Glutes Biceps Triceps Deltoids Calves	All stretches to be held for 10 seconds, except the developmental stretches which are held for 30 seconds.

Table 1.3

Eight-week fitness training plan for a person who is new to running and wants to prepare for a 10 k run:

	Week 1	Week 2	Week 3	Week 4	Week 5	Week 6	Week 7	Week 8
Mon	Rest day	Rest day	Rest day	Rest day	Rest day	Rest day	Rest day	Rest day
Tues	Run 15 mins, walk 1 to 2 mins run 15 mins	Run 15 mins, walk 1 to 2 mins, run 15 mins	Run 18 mins, walk 1 to 3 mins, run 18 mins	Run 30 mins continuously	Run 30 mins continuously	Run 30 mins continuously	Run 30 mins continuously	Run for 45 mins continuously
Wed	Flexibility class	Flexibility class	Flexibility class	Flexibility class	Flexibility class	Flexibility class	Flexibility class	Rest day
Thurs	Run 15 mins, walk 1 to 2 mins run 15 mins	Run 15 mins, walk 1 to 2 mins, run 15 mins	Run 18 mins, walk 1 to 3 mins, run 18 mins	Run 30 mins continuously	Run 30 mins continuously	Run 40 mins continuously	Run 40 mins continuously	Run for 45 mins continuously
Fri	Swim for 20 mins	Swim for 20 mins	Cycle for 20 mins	Cycle for 20 mins	Swim for 20 mins	Swim for 20 mins	Cycle for 20 mins	Rest day
Sat	Rest day	Rest day	Rest day	Rest day	Rest day	Rest day	Rest day	Rest day
Sun	Run 3 km continuously	Run 4 km continuously	Run 5 km continuously	Run 6 km continuously	Run 40 to 45 mins continuously	Run 8 km continuously	Run 50 mins continuously	Run 10 km continuously

Table 1.4

Learning aim A: Know about the components of fitness and the principles of training

Learning aim B
Explore different fitness training methods

Topic B.1 Requirements for each of the following fitness training methods

Safe, correct use of equipment

If the training equipment is not used safely or correctly, this could result in injuries. Correct equipment should be used so that the training is performed effectively.

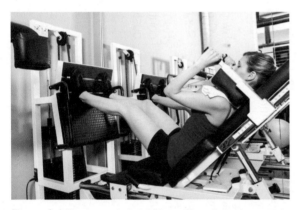

Figure 2.1 Equipment should be safe and used correctly

Safe, correct use of training technique

If the actual training technique is not carried out correctly, this can result in the training not actually providing the correct intensity or main training aim or could result in injury.

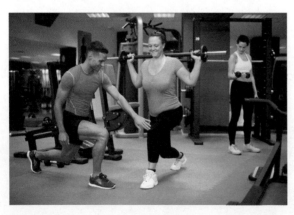

Figure 2.2 The correct training technique is important

Requirements for undertaking the fitness training method, including warm-up and cool-down

A warm-up and cool-down are essential parts of a training session. The warm-up helps to prepare the body for exercise so that there is a reduced risk of injury such as a muscle strain. Once the training session has been completed, a cool-down should be carried out to help the body recover from the exercise session, for example by helping to get rid of lactic acid and stretching out muscles.

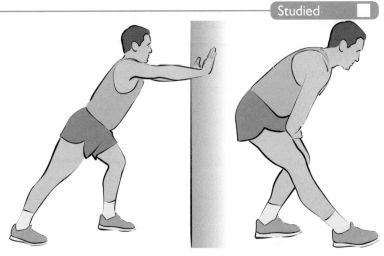

Figure 2.3 Two examples of warm-up stretches: calf stretch (left) and normal stretch (right)

Application of the basic principles of training (FITT) for each fitness training method

In order to develop a safe and effective training programme, you will need to consider the principles of training. These principles are a set of guidelines to help you understand the requirements of programme design. The principles of training are:

- **F**requency
- **I**ntensity
- **T**ime
- **T**ype.

Refer to learning aim A, page 11 for further details on each of these principles and how they can be applied to training methods.

Linking each fitness training method to the associated health-related and/or skill-related component of fitness

Different training methods can be linked to physical and skill-related components of fitness. Some training methods will link to a number of physical and skill-related components of fitness. You will need to be able to link each fitness training method to the associated health-related or skill-related component of fitness for your external assessment. This is explored in more detail in Topic B.3.

Learning aim B: Explore different fitness training methods

Topic B.2 Additional requirements for each of the fitness training methods

Advantages and disadvantages

Studied

You will need to know the advantages and disadvantages of each of the fitness tests that are carried out in this unit. Factors such as the number of people that can be tested, cost of equipment and ease of carrying out the test can all be considered. Learning aim C provides a list of advantages and disadvantages for each fitness test that you may be asked about in the external assessment.

Application of exercise intensity to fitness training methods

Studied

To ensure that specific fitness training methods, such as interval or fartlek training, are effective they need to be performed at appropriate intensities – details of how to train at the correct intensity are covered in learning aim A on page 9.

Application of principles of training to fitness training methods

Studied

This will include both the FITT principles and the additional principles of training – an example of this application can be seen in the training programmes shown in learning aim A on pages 15–17.

Appropriate application of fitness training method(s) for given situation(s)

Studied

You will need to be able to apply appropriate fitness training methods for individuals who are training for a particular sport or specific component of physical or skill-related fitness.

Appropriate application of fitness training method(s) to given client needs/goals/aims/objectives

Studied

You will need to be able to apply appropriate training methods to a specific individual who has specific targets in mind such as preparing for a competition, or improving one or more components of fitness.

Topic B.3 Fitness training methods

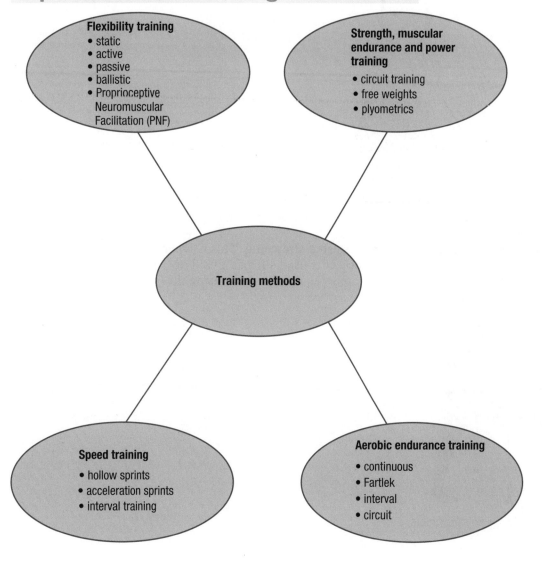

Flexibility training

Studied

There are three main types of flexibility training: static, ballistic and PNF.

Static flexibility

Static flexibility training includes active stretching and passive stretching.

Active stretching is where the performer applies internal force from another muscle group to stretch and lengthen the muscle so they are actively having to do something to produce the stretch, e.g. when you hold your arm across your body to stretch your deltoids.

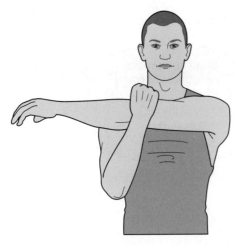

Figure 2.4 Active stretching

Passive stretching is also called assisted stretching. This is where the help of another person or an object is used such as a wall or bench. The other person/object applies external force causing the muscle to stretch.

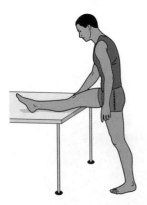

Figure 2.5 Passive stretching

Ballistic

This is where the performer carries out fast, bouncing, jerky movements through the range of motion of their joints. This type of stretching is specific to the movement pattern of the sport or activity that is to be performed. This type of stretching can cause muscle strain so it has to be carried out carefully and is usually only used in sports where the athlete already has high levels of flexibility such as gymnastics or ballet.

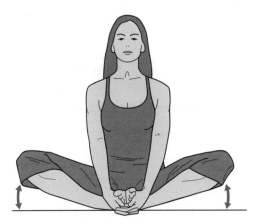

Figure 2.6 Ballistic stretching

Remember **b**allistic as **b**ouncy stretching!

Proprioceptive Neuromuscular Facilitation (PNF) technique

This type of stretching is used to develop mobility, strength and flexibility and is usually performed in the cool-down part of a training session to develop the length of the muscle. This method of stretching requires the help of a partner or an immovable object to provide resistance.

With a partner, the performer warms up and then stretches their muscle to the greatest range of their movement and then the partner helps them to hold the muscle in an isometric contraction for around 6–10 seconds. They then relax the muscle and the partner stretches the muscle further (this is static passive stretching) to allow the muscle to stretch even further.

This technique works by stopping the stretch reflex from happening.

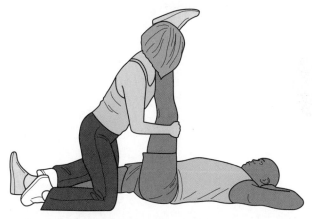

Figure 2.7 PNF stretching

Strength, muscular endurance and power training

Studied ☐

There are three main types of strength, muscular endurance and power training methods:

- circuit training
- free weights
- plyometrics.

Circuit training

This involves different stations or exercises that are all resistance based so that they can develop strength, muscular endurance and power such as using dumbbells, free weights or body weight as in press-ups. The stations or exercises are organised so that the individual going around the circuit uses different muscle groups at each station to avoid fatigue.

See Figure 2.8.

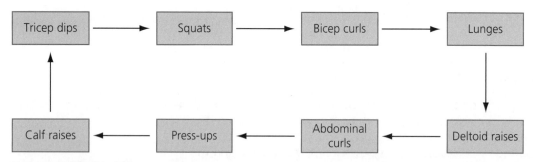

Figure 2.8 Circuit training

Free weights

A free weight is one that is not attached to machinery – examples of free weights are barbells and dumbbells.

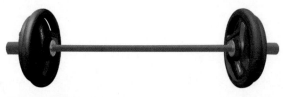

Figure 2.9 Barbell

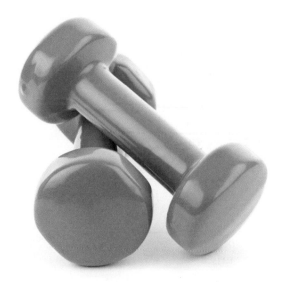

Figure 2.10 Dumbbells

These can be used to perform dynamic exercises to strengthen different muscle groups; for example, bicep curls are used to strengthen the biceps.

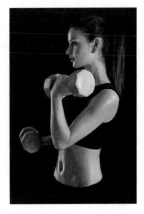

Figure 2.11

Strength, muscular endurance and power exercises

The order in which the different muscle groups are trained is important when planning strength, muscular endurance and power exercises.

Core exercises are the main resistance training lifts that use the major muscle groups of the body, such as squats that use the quadriceps and hamstrings, and the bench press which uses the chest and arms.

Assistance exercises are the exercises that use the minor muscle groups.

Core conditioning exercises are exercises that work the core muscles of the body, which include the back and the stomach in order to stabilise the spine and pelvis.

If a performer is not training for a specific sport, they will need to perform exercises which alternate between upper and lower body. If a performer is training for a specific sport, then they will concentrate their strength exercises on the muscles involved in their sport.

Intensity

The intensity is worked out as a percentage of the 1 Repetition Maximum (1 Rep Max) which is the most amount of weight that can be lifted for 1 rep. So, if a performer can lift 50 kg for 1 Rep Max in the bicep curl, 50% of their 1 Rep Max is 25 kg.

Reps and sets

The number of repetitions (reps) is one complete movement of the exercise; a set is how often you complete a group of reps. For example, you may do two sets of 10 reps on bicep curls.

Training for strength

When training for strength you should do low reps and high loads.

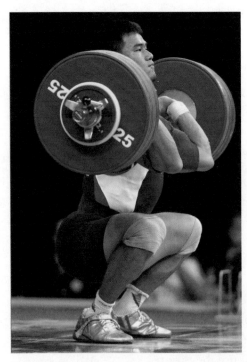

Figure 2.12

To train for maximum strength, complete 90% 1 RM and 1–6 reps.

Training for endurance

When training for endurance you should do high reps and low loads.

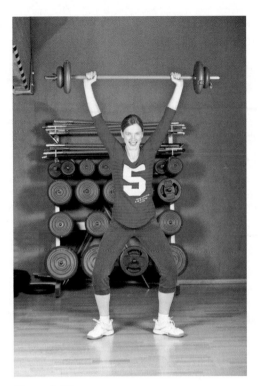

Figure 2.13

Complete 50–60% 1 RM and 20 reps.

Training for elastic strength

To train for elastic strength, complete 75% 1 RM and 12 reps.

Plyometrics

This type of training is used to develop explosive power and strength that is specific to a sport. It involves maximal lengthening (eccentric action) followed by maximal shortening (concentric action) of a muscle.

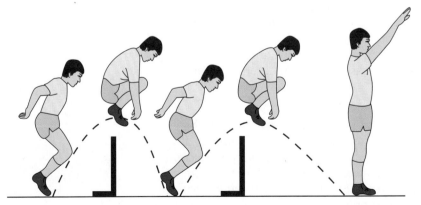

Figure 2.14

- Landing produces maximal lengthening of a muscle.
- Jumping up produces maximal shortening of a muscle.

Types of plyometric exercises include lunging, bounding, barrier hopping and jumping.

The amount of force exerted on the muscles in this type of training means that it can cause muscle soreness or injury.

This type of training is used by sports performers such as sprinters and hurdlers, and netball, volleyball and basketball players.

Aerobic endurance training

Studied ☐

There are four main types of aerobic endurance training:

- continuous
- Fartlek
- interval
- circuit.

Continuous training

This type of training requires the performer to exercise at a steady pace and moderate intensity for a minimum period of 30 minutes. For example, jogging or cycling for at least 30 minutes.

Fartlek training

In this type of training the intensity is varied by running at different speeds or over different terrain, such as up and down hills. The training is continuous with no rest periods. The use of equipment such as a harness, running with weights or running with a weighted backpack can also be used in Fartlek training to increase the intensity.

Interval training

This involves exercising followed by a rest or recovery period. The exercise time can vary from 30 seconds to five minutes followed by a recovery period which can involve complete rest or exercising at a very low intensity such as walking or light jogging. The exercise intervals will be at an intensity of around 60% of a person's maximum oxygen uptake. To increase aerobic endurance, the number of rest periods are decreased and work intensity is increased.

Circuit training

This involves different stations or exercises that are all aerobic endurance based. The exercises are performed using longer time periods and in steady rhythmical movements, usually 45 seconds work and 15 seconds rest. Exercises are chosen that work the larger muscle groups. The stations or exercises are organised so that the individual going around the circuit uses different muscle groups at each station to avoid fatigue.

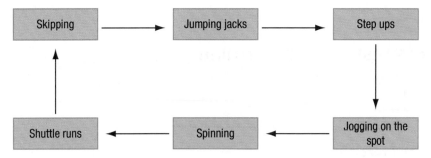
Figure 2.15 Aerobic endurance circuit training

Speed training

Studied ☐

There are three main methods for speed training:

- hollow sprints
- acceleration sprints
- interval training.

Hollow sprints

These involve a series of sprints separated by a 'hollow' period of jogging or walking between each sprint.

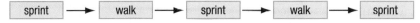

Figure 2.16 Hollow sprints

Acceleration sprints

In this type of training, the individual starts from standing or walking then increases their stride so that they then accelerate up to their maximum sprint pace. This is then followed by a rest or recovery period followed by more sprints.

Different drills can be included such as hill sprints and resistance drills using sleds, for example.

Some training methods sound the same but are used in a different way to achieve different components of fitness.

Type of training	Component of fitness and how to make training component specific	
Circuits	Strength: Resistance-based exercises	Aerobic endurance: Aerobic exercises
Free weights	Strength: High load, low reps	Muscular endurance: Low load, high reps
Interval training	Speed: Increase rest periods, increase intensity	Aerobic endurance: Decrease rest periods, decrease intensity

Table 2.1

Learning aim C
Investigate fitness testing to determine fitness levels

Topic C.1 Fitness test methods for components of fitness

Summary of fitness tests

Component of fitness	Fitness test
Flexibility	Sit and reach
Strength	Grip dynamometer
Aerobic endurance	Multi-stage fitness test Forestry step test
Speed	35-metre sprint
Speed and agility	Illinois agility run test
Anaerobic power	Vertical jump test
Muscular endurance	1-minute press-up test 1-minute sit-up test
Body composition	Body mass index (BMI) Bioelectrical impedance analysis Skinfold testing – Jackson-Pollock nomogram method

Table 3.1

You will need to know the following about each of these tests:

- What the test measures.
- The equipment required.
- How the test is carried out.
- The units that the results are measured in.
- The advantages and disadvantages of the test.
- The validity and reliability of the test.

Test name	Sit and reach test
Equipment	Sit and reach box Figure 3.1
Purpose of test	Measures the flexibility of the muscles in the lower back and hamstrings.
Protocol	1. Warm the athlete up with five minutes' jogging or cycling. 2. Ask the athlete to take off their shoes and any clothing which will limit movement. 3. The athlete sits with their legs straight and their feet against the board. Their legs and back should be straight. 4. The athlete reaches as far forward as they possibly can and pushes the marker forward. 5. Record the furthest point the marker reaches. 6. Repeat the test and record the best score.
Usually measured in	Centimetres or inches
Advantages	Quick and easy to perform. The equipment is not expensive.
Disadvantages	This test is safe to perform unless the athlete has a lower back injury, particularly a slipped disc.
Validity	This test only measures the flexibility of the lower back and hamstrings so it does not test the flexibility of all of the joints in the body.
Reliability	This depends on how much time has been spent on the warm-up. It is best to have the same warm-up before the test is taken to increase the reliability of the test. The test also has to be carried out slowly and steadily with no ballistic bouncy movements.

Table 3.2

Learning aim C: Investigate fitness testing to determine fitness levels

Test name	Grip dynamometer
Equipment	Hand grip dynamometer Figure 3.2
Purpose of test	This is a static test to assess muscular strength in the forearm and hand muscles.
Protocol	1. Adjust the handle to fit the size of your hand. 2. Hold the dynamometer in your stronger hand and keep the arm hanging by your side with the dynamometer by your thigh. 3. Squeeze the dynamometer as hard as you can for around five seconds. 4. Record the results and repeat after about a minute. 5. Take your best result.
Usually measured in	KgW
Advantages	Requires very little equipment. Quick and easy test to carry out.
Disadvantages	It only measures the strength in the forearm and hand muscles and does not give any indication of the strength of other muscle groups. The dynamometer needs to be adjusted properly for hand size; if this is not done properly the test results may not be accurate.
Validity	The test does not provide a measure of general strength as the strength of the forearms and hands does not always represent the strength of different muscle groups. If a person is right or left handed, this can affect the results – the stronger hand/arm is usually the dominant one.
Reliability	The dynamometer needs to be calibrated before use to ensure that it provides reliable data. The technique to perform the test needs to remain the same and the same rest periods between each test need to be given in order to compare results.

Table 3.3

Aerobic endurance

You will need to know the definition of aerobic endurance – it is:

The maximum amount of oxygen uptake, usually measured in ml of oxygen per kg of body mass per minute.

Test name	Forestry step test
Equipment	Bench Height for males = 40 cm Height for females = 33 cm Metronome
Purpose of test	To predict aerobic endurance levels.
Protocol	**1.** Set the metronome at 90 beats per minute. **2.** The performer stands in front of the bench then the stop watch is started and the performer starts stepping at a rate of 22.4 steps per minute in time with the metronome. **3.** Keep stepping for 5 minutes then sit down immediately. **4.** The performer finds their pulse and, after 15 seconds of sitting down, they count their pulse for 15 seconds. **5.** Use tables to work out the results for the test.
Usually measured in	ml/kg/min
Advantages	Quick and easy to perform. The equipment is not expensive. A number of people can perform the test at the same time.
Disadvantages	Different height benches are required for males and females. Taller people will find the test easier than shorter people.
Validity	Research has shown that this is a valid test to test for aerobic endurance.
Reliability	If the test protocol is followed appropriately, then the test is reliable.

Table 3.4

Learning aim C: Investigate fitness testing to determine fitness levels

Aerobic endurance

Studied ☐

Test name	Multi-stage fitness test (also known as the bleep test)
Equipment	Pre-recorded CD or tape Flat area of 20 metres Cones Tape measure
Purpose of test	Estimation of VO_2 max for aerobic endurance. VO_2 max is the maximum amount of oxygen uptake, usually measured in ml of oxygen per kg of body mass per minute.
Protocol	**1.** Mark out a length of 20 metres with cones. **2.** Start the tape; the athletes run when the first bleep sounds. They run the 20 metres before the second bleep sounds. **3.** When this bleep sounds, they turn around and run back. **4.** As they continue to do this, the time between the bleeps gets shorter and shorter so that they have to run faster and faster. **5.** If an athlete fails to get to the other end before the bleep on 3 consecutive occasions, then they are out. **6.** Record at what point the athlete dropped out. **7.** Using the table, assess the predicted VO_2 max.
Usually measured in	ml/kg/min
Advantages	This test can be used with large groups, as all the athletes will run together; the equipment is not expensive.
Disadvantages	Individuals have to be highly motivated and exercise to exhaustion in order to get appropriate data. The test is not recommended for people with health problems, injuries or low fitness levels as it is a maximal test.
Validity	The test is good for athletes whose sports require lots of running; however, for a swimmer or cyclist this test is not very valid as this test uses running to test aerobic fitness. As sport is specific, the test should involve movement in the main sport that the individual takes part in, in order to be valid.
Reliability	Running surface, climate, wind speed, if the test is performed inside or outside, motivation levels and group dynamics can all affect the reliability of the test.

Table 3.5

UNIT I Fitness for Sport and Exercise

Speed

Test name	35-metre sprint
Equipment	Flat running surface Tape measure Stop watch
Purpose of test	To measure the straight running speed of a person.
Protocol	**1.** The athlete warms up for several minutes. **2.** They then do the 35-metre run at a speed of less than their maximum. **3.** The athlete starts the test behind the line with one or two hands on the ground. **4.** The starter shouts 'go' and the athlete sprints the 35 metres as quickly as possible. **5.** This run should be repeated after 2 or 3 minutes and the average of two or three runs taken.
Usually measured in	Usually measured in seconds
Advantages	Quick and easy to perform. Does not require expensive equipment.
Disadvantages	The surface of the floor and grip of the running shoe need to be non-slip.
Validity	A valid test for sprinting speed in a straight line.
Reliability	The individual should have at least a 3-minute recovery period between each run. The timer needs to be accurate and stop the stopwatch as soon as the athlete crosses the 35-metre line.

Table 3.6

Learning aim C: Investigate fitness testing to determine fitness levels

Test name	Illinois agility run test
Equipment	Cones Stopwatch Measuring tape Flat non-slip surface Figure 3.3
Purpose of test	Test for running agility.
Protocol	1. Mark out the test with a length of 10 metres and the distance between the start and finish points being 5 metres. 2. Use four cones to mark the start, finish and the two turning points. 3. Use another four cones, spaced 3.3 metres apart down the centre. 4. The performer should lie on their front with their head to the start line and hands by their shoulders. 5. Start the stopwatch and say 'Go'. The performer gets up as quickly as possible and runs around the course without knocking the cones over, to the finish line, then stop the stopwatch.
Usually measured in	Usually measured in seconds
Advantages	Requires very little equipment, is quick and easy to administer.
Disadvantages	The test does not distinguish if the performer is better at turning right or left.
Validity	This is a valid test for sports performers who need to run and change direction in their sport such as when dodging or intercepting an opponent in football.
Reliability	The footwear and surface can affect the results of this test – if either do not provide sufficient grip, then the performer will not do so well in the test.

Table 3.7

Test name	Vertical jump test
Equipment	Wall Ruler/tape measure Chalk Figure 3.4
Purpose of test	Test of power seeing how high an athlete can jump.
Protocol	1. The athlete rubs chalk on their fingers. 2. They stand about 15 cm away from the wall. 3. With their feet flat on the floor, they reach as high as they can and make a mark on the wall. 4. The athlete then rubs more chalk on their fingers. 5. They bend their knees to 90 degrees and jump as high as they can. 6. At the top of their jump, they make a second chalk mark with their fingertips. 7. The trainer measures the difference between their two marks, this is their standing-jump score. 8. This test is best done three times so the athlete can take the best of their three jumps.
Usually measured in	kgm/s or cm
Advantages	The test is quick and easy to perform. It does not require any expensive equipment.
Disadvantages	Jumping technique can have an effect on performance rather than just the power of the legs. The test only tests for power in the legs and not upper body power.
Validity	The test is valid for measuring the power of the lower body.
Reliability	Jumping technique can affect the results – it is important that the individual has practice jumps so that improvements in power are shown in the test rather than improvements in jumping technique.

Table 3.8

Muscular endurance: arms and chest

Test name	1-minute press-up test
Equipment	Mat Stopwatch
Purpose of test	Test of muscular endurance of the arms and chest.
Protocol	1. The athlete lies in a press-up position with their back straight, toes tucked under, their elbows straight and hands shoulder width apart. 2. On the command of 'go', the athlete bends their elbows to lower their chest to the floor. 3. They return to the start position by straightening their elbows – this constitutes one repetition. 4. The athlete does as many as they can in one minute. Females can use the adapted press-up position where the knees are bent and the lower legs are in contact with the floor.
Usually measured in	Number of press-ups per minute
Advantages	Requires very little equipment; large groups can be tested at the same time.
Disadvantages	Only tests for the endurance of the arms and the chest. The test requires high levels of motivation so that the maximum number of repetitions are completed.
Validity	This is a good test for muscular endurance but is only specific to the chest and the arms.
Reliability	The test requires high levels of motivation so the individuals must be highly motivated to attain reliable results. The tester needs to ensure that the press-ups are carried out using the correct technique.

Table 3.9

Muscular endurance: abdominals

Test name	1-minute sit-up test
Equipment	Mat Stopwatch
Purpose of test	Test of muscular endurance of the abdominals.
Protocol	1. The athlete lies on the floor with their fingers on their temples and their knees bent. 2. On the command of 'go', the athlete sits up until their elbows touch their knees. 3. They return to the start position with the back of their head touching the floor. This constitutes one repetition. 4. The athlete does as many as they can in 1 minute.
Usually measured in	Number of sit-ups per minute
Advantages	Requires very little equipment; large groups can be tested at the same time.
Disadvantages	Only tests for endurance of the abdominals. The test requires high levels of motivation so that the maximum number of repetitions are completed.
Validity	A full sit-up also uses the hip flexor muscles so the test also tests the muscular endurance of the hip flexor muscles as well as the abdominals.
Reliability	The test does rely on high levels of motivation so the individuals must be highly motivated to attain reliable results.

Table 3.10

Learning aim C: Investigate fitness testing to determine fitness levels

Body composition

Test name	Body Mass Index (BMI)
Equipment	Weighing scales Stadiometer
Purpose of test	To work out if a person is overweight.
Protocol	BMI = Weight (kg)/ (Height (m) x Height (m))
Usually measured in	kg/m^2
Advantages	Requires very little equipment. It is a quick and easy test to perform. The individual does not have to remove any clothing so it is less embarrassing than the skinfold test.
Disadvantages	This test can be used for the average adult but cannot be used for pregnant women, children, very muscular athletes or people over the age of 60.
Validity	It does not take into account the actual body composition: a person may have a lot of muscle tissue and very little body fat but still gain a score of being overweight/fat on the BMI. The test does not actually measure body composition.
Reliability	As long as body weight and body height are measured correctly, the test is reliable.

Table 3.11

You will need to know how to work out a person's BMI from their weight (in kilograms) and height (in metres).

For example:

A person is 152 cm tall and weighs 56 kg – what is their BMI?

$$BMI = 56/1.52^2$$

$$= 56/2.31$$

$$= 24$$

Always show your working out – you may get extra marks for this!

Bioelectrical impedance analysis test

See Table 3.12 for an outline of this test.

This test works because fat-free tissues such as muscle and bone are good conductors of electrical current and fat is not a good conductor. The amount of resistance to the electrical current is related to the amount of fat-free tissue in the body and so can be used to estimate percentage body fat.

Test name	Bioelectrical Impedance Analysis (BIA)
Equipment	Bioelectrical Impedance Analysis Analyser Alcohol pads Weighing scales Tape measure or other means of measuring height Electrodes placed on the right hand and right foot Detection electrode Current source electrode Figure 3.5
Purpose of test	Used for prediction of percentage body fat.
Protocol	1. Remove the shoe and sock on the right foot. 2. The individual should lie on a bed or a mat and have their right hand and right foot swabbed with an alcohol wipe. 3. Electrodes are placed on the right hand and right foot with their legs and arms away from their body. 4. A very small electrical current is passed through the body.
Usually measured in	Percentage body fat
Advantages	The individual does not have to remove any clothing so it is not as embarrassing as the skinfold test.
Disadvantages	The equipment is quite expensive. The individual also has to ensure that they are hydrated and have not drunk alcohol 48 hours prior to the test or taken part in high intensity exercise 12 hours prior to the test. A person with a pacemaker or a pregnant woman should not be tested using this equipment.
Validity	It is not as accurate as skinfold measurements. The scores are influenced by how well hydrated a person is. If a person is dehydrated, their body fat is overestimated.
Reliability	The individual must be properly hydrated prior to the test and have followed all the pre-test guidelines to ensure the results are reliable.

Table 3.12

Body composition

Test name	Skinfold testing via the Jackson-Pollock nomogram method
Equipment	Skinfold callipers Figure 3.6
Purpose of test	Prediction of percentage body fat.
Protocol	Sites for males: chest, abdomen and thigh. Sites for females: triceps, suprailiac and thigh. 1. Take the measurements on the right side of the body. 2. Mark the client up accurately. 3. Pinch the skin 1 cm above the marked site. 4. Pull the fat away from the muscle. 5. Place the callipers halfway between the top and bottom of the skinfold. 6. Allow the callipers to settle for 1–2 seconds. 7. Take the reading and wait 15 seconds before repeating for accuracy. 8. Add up the total of the three measurements in mm. 9. Plot the age of the individual and the sum of the three skinfolds (mm) on the nomogram. 10. Use a ruler to join up the two plots – percentage body fat can be seen where the two lines cross over the percentage body fat lines to the closest 0.5%, according to gender.

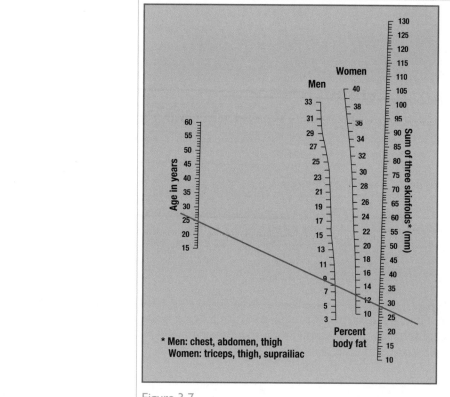

Figure 3.7

Usually measured in	Percentage body fat
Advantages	It provides a good estimation of the body fat of a person.
Disadvantages	The person being tested has to remove or adjust their clothing and have parts of their body 'pinched' by the test, which can be embarrassing.
Validity	This is one of the most valid tests for estimating body fat percentage.
Reliability	The body parts must be tested in the same places in order to get reliable results, this relies to some extent on the skill of the tester to accurately and consistently identify the sites.

Table 3.13

Topic C.2 Importance of fitness testing to sports performers and coaches

Monitoring/improving performance

Studied ☐

Fitness tests are used by sports performers and coaches to give baseline data for monitoring/improving performance.

Designing training programmes

Studied ☐

Fitness tests are taken regularly to monitor if a training programme is producing the desired results. Training programmes can be changed or modified depending on the results from the fitness tests.

Goal setting

Studied ☐

The results can also give a performer something to aim for and help them with their goal setting – for example, they may want to achieve level 15 on the multi-stage fitness test in their next fitness test.

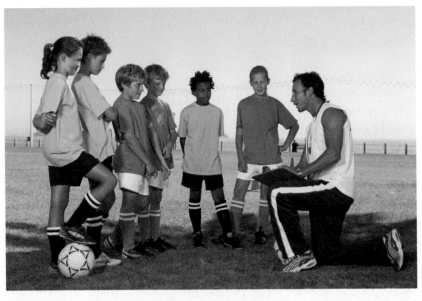

Figure 3.8

Topic C.3 Requirements for administration of each fitness test

When carrying out the fitness tests listed above, it is important to consider the following factors.

Pre-test procedures

Studied

When testing athletes, it is important that the tests are safe and that the conditions the tests are performed in are consistent and stable. The athlete should:

- Have medical clearance for any health conditions.
- Be free of injuries.
- Be wearing appropriate clothing.
- Not have had a heavy meal three hours before the test.
- Have had a good night's sleep.
- Not have trained on the day and be fully recovered from previous training.
- Have avoided stimulants such as tea, coffee or nicotine for two hours before the test.

The area where the tests are performed should be:

- At room temperature (around 18 degrees Celsius).
- Well ventilated.
- Clean and dust-free.

Medical referral

An athlete should not be tested and should be referred to the doctor if they are experiencing any of the following:

- muscle injuries
- chest pain or tightness
- light-headedness or dizziness
- irregular or rapid pulse
- joint pain
- headaches
- shortness of breath.

These safety procedures are very important. It is valuable to get good results but not at the cost of an athlete's health. It is also important to check that the athlete does not get any symptoms after the test has been conducted.

Informed consent

An informed consent form makes the athlete aware of what is involved in the exercise testing and any risks there may be. They

Learning aim C: Investigate fitness testing to determine fitness levels

can then give their agreement or consent to undertake the tests with an awareness of the risks which are involved. It provides documented evidence that shows that participants have been provided with all the necessary information to undertake the test. The informed consent form confirms that the individual:

- is able to follow the test method
- knows exactly what is required of them during testing
- has fully consented to their participation in the fitness tests
- knows that they are able to ask any questions relating to the tests
- understands that they can withdraw from the test at any time.

The consent form should be signed and dated by the participant, the tester and by a tutor if you are performing the tests at school or college. If the participant is under 18 years of age, a parent or guardian will also be required to give their consent for participation.

Calibration of equipment

This is the process of checking (and if necessary adjusting) the accuracy of fitness testing equipment before it is used, by comparing it to a recognised standard. Prior to testing, equipment should be checked carefully. If equipment is not correctly calibrated it could lead to inaccurate (invalid) results.

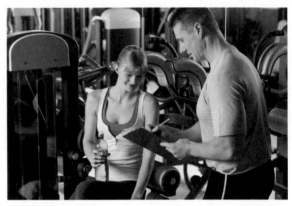

Figure 3.9 Participants in fitness tests should give their informed consent

Knowledge of standard test methods and equipment/resources required

Studied ▢

In order to carry out a test correctly and safely, it is important that you have an understanding of published standard test methods and the equipment and resources needed to carry out the test. Details of the methods and equipment needed for each individual fitness test are provided in the 'protocol' and 'equipment' rows of the tables in Topic C.1.

Purpose of each fitness test

Studied ▢

It is also essential to know the purpose of each fitness test. This will help you to select an appropriate test to measure the component of fitness you are trying to test. For example, if you are trying to measure percentage of body fat, you will need to know that this is the purpose of skinfold testing in order to make sure you select that fitness test.

Accurate measurement and recording of test results

Studied ☐

You should ensure that you measure and record test results accurately so that you can draw conclusions from them and analyse and evaluate the results.

Processing of test results for interpretation

You should be able to compare the results from your fitness test with published data tables so that you can interpret the results of your test – is your athlete's performance good, average or below average when compared with others' results? It is important to use appropriate units when comparing data. For example, if you have measured results for a 35 m sprint test in seconds, you need to make sure that published data is also measured in seconds so that comparison is possible and meaningful.

Safely selecting an appropriate test

Studied ☐

It is important to select a test that is appropriate and safe for your athlete to carry out. For example, a Bioelectrical Impedance Analysis should not be carried out by anyone who has drunk alcohol 48 hours prior to the test or taken part in high intensity exercise 12 hours prior to the test. A person with a pacemaker or a pregnant woman should not be tested using this equipment. It is important to have knowledge of a person's health before carrying out a test so you can ensure they do not carry out a test that is inappropriate or dangerous for them.

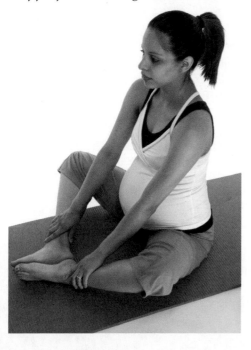

Figure 3.10 Ensure the test is appropriate, for example, pregnant women should not take the bioelectrical impedance analysis

Reliability, validity and practicality

Studied ☐

Fitness tests need to be valid and reliable to provide useful data. The terms can be understood by asking the following questions:

- Validity – Does the test actually test for the component of fitness that it says it is testing? For example, a speed test using shuttle runs may actually test the athlete's ability to turn to a greater extent than their actual speed so it will not be a valid test for speed.
- Reliability – If the test is repeated do you get the same results?
- Practicality – This is to do with whether the test can actually be carried out for the person or people it is intended for and includes considering the number of people that need to be tested, the equipment and resources available etc.

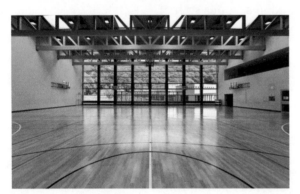

Figure 3.11 The environment you conduct your test in may impact the results

- The conditions of the test must always be identical so that it is likely that the same results will be produced – this includes not only the temperature and the environment but also the equipment to ensure that it is calibrated and working properly. Two testers may also get different results when they perform a test, such as the skinfold test. These factors all have to be taken in to account so that any changes in the test results are due to changes in the fitness of the performer taking part in the test and not due to errors in the measurements.

Advantages and disadvantages of fitness test methods

Studied ☐

You should also know the advantages and disadvantages of each test method to help you make an assessment of whether a test is appropriate. Details of the advantages and disadvantages for each individual fitness test are provided in the tables in Topic C.1.

Topic C.4 Interpretation of fitness test results

For the external assessment, you will need to be able to:

Compare fitness test results to normative published data

You will need to be able to find your score on the fitness table and find out what that score means, for example average, good, poor compared to other people.

Compare fitness test results to those of peers

You need to compare your results with others taking the fitness test – did you get higher or lower results than other people in your class for each fitness test?

Draw conclusions from data results

Did your results show that you need to improve some components of fitness?

Analyse and evaluate test results

You will need to be able to explain why you and other people got the results you did. For example, if you take part in lots of flexibility exercises such as yoga then you will probably get a high score on the sit and reach test.

Suggest and justify appropriate recommendations for improvements to fitness for a given purpose/situation/participant

You will need to be able to compare your results to the normative data and work out which components of fitness you need to improve on in comparison to the other fitness test results. For example, if you had high scores in aerobic endurance, speed and power but very low scores in flexibility, then you will need to improve your flexibility training as having low levels of flexibility can lead to muscle strains and so on.

External assessment: Question paper 1

1. Omar is a lightweight boxer. He has applied the principles of training to his programme to ensure his performance increases.

Which principle of training is Omar applying when he carries out boxing practice punching a punch bag? (1)

(a) Progression ☐

(b) Specificity ☐

(c) Adaptation ☐

(d) Reversibility ☐

2. Using a variety of different fitness training methods is a good way to prevent boredom and to keep sports people interested in training. One method of fitness training is shown in the photograph below.

What fitness training method is being performed? (1)

(a) PNF ☐

(b) Circuit Training ☐

(c) Free weights ☐

(d) Plyometrics ☐

3. Max is an athlete. He belongs to a local athletics club and is using training methods to increase his fitness and performance.

Which component of fitness will hollow sprints help to develop? (1)

(a) Agility ☐

(b) Speed ☐

(c) Flexibility ☐

(d) Muscular endurance ☐

4. Use the words below to complete the blanks. (2)

.... is having an adequate range of motion in all joints of the body.

Flexibility

Agility

Bone

Joints

5. It is important to follow the FITT principles of training when developing a fitness training programme. Specificity is one of the additional principles of training. Name two other additional principles of training. (2)

Write your answers in the box below.

6. Identify the types of training described below. Write your answers in the boxes provided.

(a) This type of training is usually done at a constant and steady pace with no rest periods. (1)

(b) This type of training involves periods of high-intensity work followed by short rest periods.(1)

7. Exercise intensity is important for a training programme. Exercise intensity can use target zones to work out how hard a person should be exercising.

(a) What is meant by the term 'target zone'? **(1)**

(b) How is the target zone calculated? **(2)**

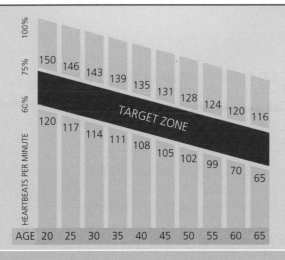

8. It is very important that sports activities are made safe. Safety precautions must be followed to ensure that the sport is as safe as possible for everyone who is involved in the activity.

(a) Suggest a safety precaution which sports players must consider before taking part in a named activity. **(2)**

(b) Explain two possible outcomes of not carrying out these safety aspects. **(2)**

9. Aerobic endurance is a component of fitness. The components of fitness are important to a sports person. If they know which ones are needed for their sports, they can train that component to ensure that their level of fitness is high.

Which of the following is another name for aerobic endurance? (1)

(a) Muscular fitness ☐

(b) Muscular endurance ☐

(c) Aerobic power ☐

(d) Aerobic fitness ☐

10. The cardiorespiratory system plays a very important role in the ability of a performer to be able to compete at their best for as long as possible.

Describe the role of the cardiorespiratory system. (3)

11. The body will adapt to the extra demands that training puts on the different body systems so that fitness increases. Training must be continuously increased to higher levels to ensure that progress is made.

Discuss how this might be done to ensure that the body systems adapt to cope with higher levels of exercise. Refer to a sport of your choice to develop your answer. (8)

12. Fitness testing is very important to a sports person as it lets them know what level they are at and where they need to improve. Fitness testing can identify their strengths and weaknesses.
James is taking part in a fitness test.

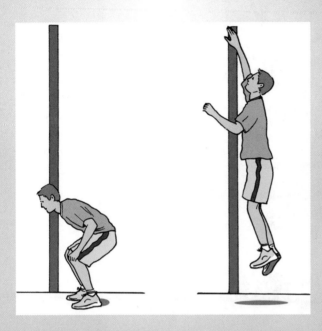

(a) What is this fitness test that James is participating in called? (1)

Write your answer in the box below.

(b) Which component of James's fitness is this test measuring? (1)

Write your answer in the box below.

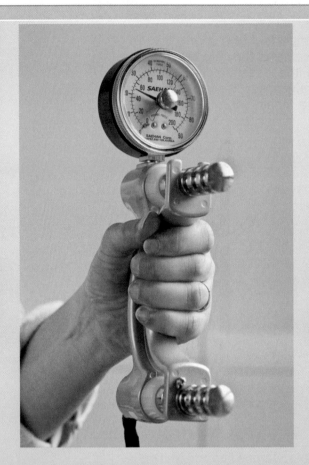

Colin is taking part in a fitness test.

(c) What is the fitness test that Colin is participating in called? **(1)**

Write your answer in the box below.

(d) Which component of Colin's fitness is this test measuring? **(1)**

Write your answer in the box below.

13. Nadia is using strength training exercises to increase her muscular strength.

(a) Explain why it is important that strength training exercises should be followed by stretching. (2)

(b) Explain a method used to test flexibility. (4)

14. Marc wants to increase his strength so that he can perform better in his chosen sports. He is developing a strength-training programme to follow in training sessions.

(a) Describe the key features of a weight-training programme Marc could use to build up his strength. (2)

(b) Name two sports for which strength training would be relevant. (2)

15. Aerobics fitness is very important to sports people. This component of fitness enables them to keep going for longer. For example, aerobic fitness is what allows a footballer to keep going throughout the entire length of a football match.

Other than playing football, name another sports activity which could improve cardiovascular fitness. (1)

16. When carrying out fitness tests it is very important that the tests are carried out reliably so that the results obtained can be said to be valid.

Explain how you can ensure that you carry out a fitness test reliably. (4)

17. Katie is carrying out fitness tests on her hockey team. She has been using different pieces of equipment.

(a) What is the name of the piece of fitness testing equipment in the photograph below? **(1)**

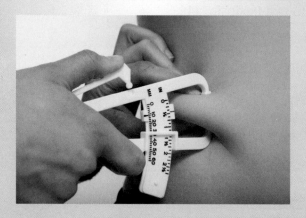

(b) Identify which test this piece of equipment could be used for. **(1)**

18. It is important that fitness test results can be compared to standard or normative data. Ryan has been using the sit and reach test to measure his flexibility.

(a) Identify the units that are used to measure the sit and reach test. **(1)**

(b) Ryan took the sit and reach test and scored 8.2. Using the table below, identify what level of fitness this score indicates Ryan has for flexibility. **(1)**

Gender	Excellent	Above average	Average	Below average	Poor
Male	>14	14.0–11.0	10.9–7.0	6.9–4.0	<4
Female	>15	15.0–12.0	11.9–7.0	6.9–4.0	<4

External assessment: Question paper 2

1. Chris is interested in training for a marathon and has been advised that he should do continuous training to prepare for it.

Which of the FITT principles does this advice relate to? (1)

(a) frequency ☐

(b) intensity ☐

(c) time ☐

(d) type ☐

2. One component of fitness needed for a sprinter is reaction time. Explain how reaction time can lead to a sprinter being successful.

Write your answer in the box below. (3)

3. The 1-minute sit-up test can be used to assess muscular endurance. Explain two advantages and two disadvantages of this test.

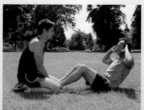

Write your answer in the box below. (4)

4.

(a) What type of training is being performed in the picture? (1)

(i) resistance ☐

(ii) fartlek ☐

(iii) plyometrics ☐

(iv) circuit ☐

(b) What component of fitness will this type of training improve? (1)

(i) flexibility ☐

(ii) aerobic endurance ☐

(iii) muscular endurance ☐

(iv) agility ☐

5. Complete the following definitions. (2)

...............................: The ability of a sports performer to quickly and precisely move or change direction without losing balance or time.
...............................: The product of strength and speed.

AGILITY   POWER   BALANCE   REACTION TIME   STRENGTH

6.

(a) Describe what is meant by the term 'variation' when planning training programmes. Write your answer in the box below. **(1)**

(b) Explain why variation is an important principle of training. Write your answer in the box below. **(1)**

7. Callum is 18 and wants to improve his cardiovascular fitness. He has been told to train at between 60% and 85% of his maximum heart rate.

(a) What are the lower and upper limits of his 'training range' to the nearest whole number? Show your working in the box below. **(3)**

(b) Explain the approximate rating of perceived exertion at the upper limit of this training range. Write your answer in the box below. **(2)**

8. In a resistance training session, exercises should be performed in a particular order. Which of the following would be an example of the correct order of exercises? **(1)**

(a) calf raise, squat, bicep curl, seated row ☐

(b) squat, seated row, calf raise, bicep curl ☐

(c) bicep curl, calf raise, squat, seated row ☐

(d) seated row, bicep curl, calf raise, squat ☐

9. In resistance training athletes will perform 'repetitions' and 'sets'. Identify the meaning of these terms. **(2)**

REPETITION

[blank box]

SETS

[blank box]

10. Which of the following training methods cannot be used to improve aerobic endurance? **(1)**

(a) fartlek ☐

(b) interval ☐

(c) circuit ☐

(d) plyometrics ☐

11. Fitness testing helps to identify training needs and monitor an athlete's progress. The image below shows a piece of fitness testing equipment.

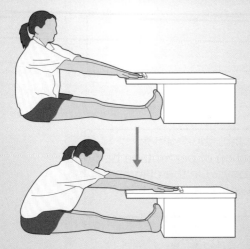

(a) What is the name of this test? **(1)**

(b) What component of fitness does it assess? **(1)**

(c) Describe one factor that could affect the validity and one factor that could affect the reliability of the test. **(2)**

12. Body composition can be measured in different ways. Identify three ways of measuring body composition. Write your answer in the box below. **(3)**

13. The skinfold locations in the Jackson-Pollock nomogram method for prediction of percentage body fat are different for girls and boys. On the diagrams below identify where the measurements are taken for males and females. **(2)**

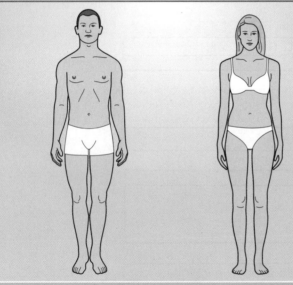

14. Robert would like to take part in a personal fitness programme to improve his muscular strength. Describe the factors that would have to be considered when planning his fitness programme.

Write your answers in the box below. **(8)**

15. Samira is 20 and is a 1500 m runner. She has taken the multi-stage fitness test and achieved a level of 10.8.

(a) Using the conversion chart, what is her predicted VO$_2$ max score? **(1)**

Level	Shuttle	VO$_2$ Max
9	4	44.5
9	6	45.2
9	8	45.8
9	11	46.8
10	2	47.4
10	4	48.0
10	6	48.7
10	8	49.3
10	11	50.2

(b) Using the information provided in the table, interpret her VO$_2$ max score. **(1)**

Age	Very Poor	Poor	Fair	Good	Excellent	Superior
13-19	<25.0	25.0-30.9	31.0-34.9	35.0-38.9	39.0-41.9	>41.9
20-29	<23.6	23.6-28.9	29.0-32.9	33.0-36.9	37.0-41.0	>41.0
30-39	<22.8	22.8-26.9	27.0-31.4	31.5-35.6	35.7-40.0	>40.0
40-49	<21.0	21.0-24.4	24.5-28.9	29.0-32.8	32.9-36.9	>36.9
50-59	<20.2	20.2-22.7	22.8-26.9	27.0-31.4	31.5-35.7	>35.7
60+	<17.5	17.5-20.1	20.2-24.4	24.5-30.2	30.3-31.4	>31.4

(c) What are the units of measurement for VO$_2$? **(1)**

    (i) ml/kg/min
    (ii) kg/m2
    (iii) kgm/s
    (iv) kg/W

16. The picture shows an athlete performing a sports specific training method. Name the specific training method. **(1)**

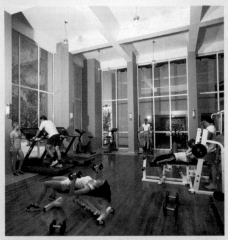

17. Angus is training for a weightlifting competition and wants to improve his maximum muscular strength. His one rep max for the squat is 150 kg. Complete the following table to provide him with the specifics of his session. **(3)**

Exercise	1 RM	Reps	Sets	Weight
Squat	150 kg			

18. Explain the importance of fitness testing to sports performers and coaches.

Write your answer in the box below. **(3)**

Unit 2
Practical Sports Performance

Unit 2, Practical Sports Performance, is an internally assessed, compulsory unit with three learning aims:

- Learning aim A: Understand the rules, regulations and scoring systems for selected sports
- Learning aim B: Practically demonstrate skills, techniques and tactics in selected sports
- Learning aim C: Be able to review sports performance.

In this unit you will develop your practical sports performance through taking part in activities and reviewing your performance and the performance of others. By observing sports officials you will develop your understanding of the rules and regulations of various sports in learning aim A. In learning aim B you will have the opportunity to take part in a number of different sports and will need to show skills, techniques and tactics in your chosen sport. Learning aim C asks you to review your performance in your chosen sports, consider your strengths and weaknesses and think about plans to develop your performance.

Each learning aim is divided in to two sections. The first section focuses on the content of the learning aim and each of the topics are covered. At the end of each learning aim there are some knowledge recap questions to test your understanding of the subject. The answers for the knowledge recap questions can be found at the end of the book.

The second section of each learning aim provides support with assessment by using evidence generated by a student, for each grading criterion, with feedback from an assessor. The assessor has highlighted where the evidence is sufficient to satisfy the grading criterion and provided developmental feedback when additional work is required.

At the end of the book is an example of an assignment brief for this unit. The sample assignment brief contains tasks that would allow you to generate the evidence needed to meet all the assessment criteria in the unit. The assessment criteria are also outlined in a table following the brief.

Learning aim A
Understand the rules, regulations and scoring systems for selected sports

Assessment criteria

2A.P1 Describe the rules, regulations and scoring systems of two selected sports.

2A.P2 Apply the rules of a selected sport in four specific situations.

2A.P3 Describe the roles and responsibilities of officials from two selected sports.

2A.M1 For each of the two selected sports, explain the roles and responsibilities of officials and the application of rules, regulations and scoring systems.

2A.D1 Compare and contrast the roles and responsibilities of officials from two selected sports, suggesting valid recommendations for improvements to the application of rules, regulations and scoring systems for each sport.

Topic A.1 Rules (or laws)

Rules are a set of agreed standards that are laid down to standardise how a sport is to be played, such as how many people are on each side and how you score points. Rules also cover what behaviour is acceptable and unacceptable and how unacceptable behaviour can be punished. Rules are set down by national or international governing bodies of sport, such as FIFA (football) or the IRB (rugby union). In some sports, such as cricket, the rules are referred to as 'laws'.

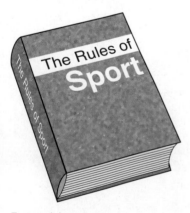

Figure 4.1

Governing body of sport

The governing body of a sport is represented by the group of people who agree the rules and appoint officials to implement them, e.g. the FA (football) and the RFL (rugby football league).

Governing bodies can be international and they agree rules for sports played in all countries; they also organise competitions. In the UK, National Governing Bodies ensure these international rules are implemented in all forms of a sport. They are also responsible for organising sporting competitions in the UK.

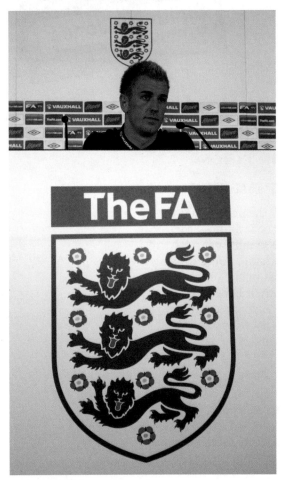

Figure 4.2

Topic A.2 Regulations

Regulations relate to specific aspects of the rules and how the rule should be implemented. Regulations include details of various elements, including the playing surface; the type of equipment that is acceptable, for example, what any equipment is made from, length of studs; any timing regulations such as time outs or added on time; methods of substituting players; health and safety and officials.

Topic A.3 Scoring systems

The scoring system is the method a sport uses to decide who the winner is. The simplest scoring systems are where a point is recorded for each goal, such as in football or hockey. Athletics, which uses times or distances, also has an easy to understand method of deciding who the winner is. Some sports such as golf, rugby and tennis have complex scoring methods. These sports all have scoring methods that are clear and are not based on the opinion of judges or officials. Some sports, such as diving, gymnastics, ice skating, boxing and synchronised swimming, have scoring systems that are based on the opinions of the officials who have been appointed to judge the sport. This can lead to some controversial decisions that not all the people watching the sport may agree with.

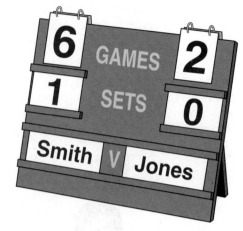

Figure 4.3

Topic A.4 Application of the rules/laws of sports in different situations

It is the officials' role to apply the rules/laws to the action that they are watching. For example, in football the referee will blow their whistle if they see foul play and the referee's assistant will raise their flag if they judge that a player has been offside. Some officials have many rules to apply. For example, umpires in cricket have to judge whether a player is out LBW, run out or their bat has made contact with the ball. In cricket and tennis, the players are able to appeal a decision that an official has made and these sports use technology to help them make accurate decisions.

Topic A.5 Sports

There is a range of sports that could be considered as part of this learning aim, for example, cricket, hockey, netball, rounders, volleyball, wheelchair basketball, golf, trampolining, table tennis, archery, judo, cross-country running, Boccia, fencing, orienteering, skiing, canoeing, sailing and mountain biking. Each sport has different rules, regulations and scoring systems, and the roles and responsibilities of the officials will vary from sport to sport.

Topic A.6 Roles of officials

Officials are the people or groups of people who ensure that the participants play to the rules and regulations of a sport. They may also be responsible for time-keeping, starting play and scoring.

Some of these officials are positioned on the field of play, such as football referees or cricket umpires; some are close to the play, such as tennis umpires or boxing judges; and some are further away from the action, such as officials in cycling or gymnastics.

Officials are also called umpires, referees or judges.

The roles of officials are the duties they have to perform in enforcing the rules of the sport. For example, in football a referee is in charge of the game and enforcing the rules; the referee's assistants and the fourth official are there to assist the referee in implementing the rules.

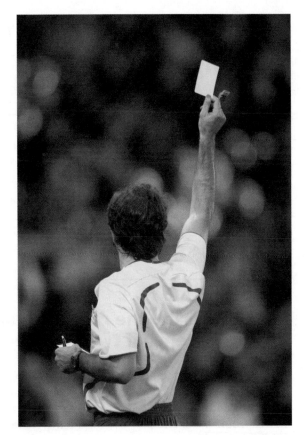

Figure 4.4

Topic A.7 Responsibilities of officials

The responsibilities of officials describe how they implement these rules, for example, punishing foul play, controlling players and ensuring they are wearing the correct equipment. The health and safety of all participants is the responsibility of officials.

Officials communicate in different ways: by speaking and listening to players, using their whistle to stop play and hand signals to convey their decisions. In some sporting situations, officials can rely on technology; for example, a tennis or cricket umpire can use 'Hawkeye' to review decisions.

Knowledge recap

1. Describe what is meant by the rules of a sport.

2. Identify two things a governing body does.

3. Identify three roles of umpires in tennis.

Assessment guidance for learning aim A

Scenario

You have been offered a job in your local sports centre to help run a summer holiday sports scheme for the children aged 11–13. The sports centre is able to offer the children the opportunity to play a variety of sports, but for many of them it will be the first time they have played some of the sports. The manager of the scheme has asked you to complete several activities that will help the children to participate in the sports.

2A.P1 ## Describe the rules, regulations and scoring systems of two selected sports

Assessor report: The command verb in the grading criterion is **describe**. In the answer we would expect to see a detailed account of the rules, regulations and scoring systems, to the extent that a person reading the answer would be able to play or officiate the game in line with the rules and regulations.

✍ Learner answer

Rules

Sport 1 – Badminton

- To win a game, it's the first to 21 points.
- To win the match you need to win the best of three games.
- When you lose a point, the serve is changed to your opponent.
- If the score is 20–20, the game is won by the player who scores two consecutive points.
- If the game gets to 29–29, the player who gets to 30 points wins the game.
- The net is 5 feet high.
- The player who wins a game takes the first serve of the next match.
- If a player fails with their serve, it's a point to the opposition.

- You are not allowed to reach over the net to play the shuttlecock.
- Before a game you toss a coin to decide who serves first and which end you play from.
- If the shuttlecock lands on a line it counts as in.
- If a shuttlecock hits a player they lose the point.
- The first serve of a game is taken from the right-hand side of the court.
- The serve must be done from below waist height.

Sport 2 – Handball

The playing court

- Court measures 20 metres by 40 metres and there is a goal line at 6 metres.
- The goal is 2 metres by 3 metres.
- Players may jump into the goal area if they release the ball before landing.

The ball

- Handball is played with a 32-panel leather ball.
- For women the ball weighs 325–400 grams and for men 425–475 grams.

Number of players

- There are seven players on each team.
- Of these seven players, six are court players and one the goalkeeper.
- A maximum of 12 players may participate in the game.

Referees

- There are two referees.
- They are the court referee and the goal line referee.

Length of game

- For players aged over 18, the game consists of two, 30-minute halves with 10 minutes half-time.

Scoring

- A goal is scored when the whole of the ball has crossed the goal line on the inside of the goal.

Playing the ball

- A player can hold the ball for a maximum of 3 seconds.
- A player can take a maximum of three steps before dribbling the ball.

Defending

- A player may use their torso to obstruct an opponent with or without the ball.
- A player cannot use an outstretched arm to push, hold or trip an opponent.
- An attacking player cannot charge into a defensive player.

Assessor report: The candidate has completed the rules of badminton in a brief way. To gain P1 they would need to cover the rules in more detail and give details of the dimensions of the playing area and the numbers of officials involved. It is also a good idea to bunch together the rules relating to different aspects of the game, such as the serve. The work on the scoring system, although strictly speaking they are rules, would be better left for the section on scoring systems. The work on handball is excellent. It covers all the main rules and puts them in logical groups and in a logical order. A similar approach should be adopted for the work on badminton.

Regulations

In badminton there are regulations regarding the equipment and the court. The racket should measure 2.5 feet long and be 8 inches wide. Players cannot attach anything to their racket. The shuttlecock will consist of 16 feathers attached to a cork base; it should weigh less than half an ounce. The net should be 4 feet off the ground and be of a white colour with a white strip across the top. The court needs to be kept dry and the court lines need to be marked in white paint.

In handball the team can name five substitutes and a substitute can be used at any time through the substitution area as long as the player being replaced has left the court. The court must be kept dry and have clearly marked lines on it. There must be benches for substitutes. The court must be checked before a game and all players must be checked to ensure they are not wearing jewellery and are wearing appropriate clothing and footwear.

Assessor report: These regulations have been covered well. It can be difficult to differentiate between rules and regulations, but the regulations regarding clothing and equipment are well covered. There is an opportunity here to cover detail about the badminton court, its dimensions and the requirements for space around and above the court. There are some factual inaccuracies given here about the height of the net off the ground and its colour.

Scoring systems

Badminton

A match is three games long and consists of three games; the winner is the first to two games.

To win a game, you have to get to 21 points before your opponent, but you have to be at least two points clear to win.

You will win a point if:

- The shuttlecock hits the floor on your opponent's side.
- Your opponent hits the shuttlecock into the net.
- Your opponent hits the shuttlecock outside the lines of the court.
- The shuttlecock hits your opponent.

Handball

A goal is scored when the entire ball crosses the goal line inside the goal. A goal may be scored from a free throw, a throw in, throw off or a goal throw. The team who scores the most goals wins the match.

Assessor report: The information on scoring in handball is quite straightforward but more detail could be provided on badminton, such as what happens at 20–20 and how many points they play for.

Assessor report – overall

What is good about this assessment evidence?

The candidate has produced good descriptions of the rules, regulations and scoring systems of two sports.

What could be improved about this assessment evidence?

The organisation of the work could be improved so that the work is grouped under headings and subheadings. The learner also needs to make sure there are no factual inaccuracies in the information they provide for both sports.

(2A.P2) Apply the rules of a selected sport in four specific situations

✎ **Learner answer**

I play handball for a local team and have used one of our practice sessions to show that I can apply the rules of handball.

My coach has completed the observation statements.

Assessor report: The command verb for 2B.P2 is to **apply** the rules of a selected sport. The learner needs to show in practice that they can take the rules of a sport and accurately apply them to a game situation where they are active as an official.

The learner has clearly identified a situation where they will able to achieve the grading criterion and a credible witness who can confirm that they have applied the criterion.

✎ **Learner answer**

I have attached the observation document from my teacher.

OBSERVATION RECORD	
Learner name:	Stephen Patrick
Assessor name:	Anne Coates
Qualification:	Edexcel BTEC Level 2 First Award in Sport
Unit:	Practical Sports Performance
Description of activity and grading criterion	
2A.P2 – Apply the rules of a selected sport in four specific situations	
Stephen is acting as an official in a handball match between two teams of his peers in a practical sports session. I was the other official for the match.	
What the learner did	
Stephen acted as one of the officials and applied the rules of handball in a range of situations.	

How the learner met the requirements of the grading criterion			
11\09\2012 – Stephen was able to show that he could he could apply the rules of handball in a range of situations. Stephen penalised a player who held the ball for over 3 seconds without passing it to a team mate. He correctly awarded a free-throw to the opposition. Stephen penalised a player who took more than three steps before passing the ball. He correctly awarded a free-throw to the opposition. Stephen penalised a defending player who used an outstretched arm to deny a player a shot on goal. He correctly awarded a seven-meter throw and gave the offending player a warning. Stephen penalised an attacking player who charged into a defending player to create a goal scoring chance. He correctly awarded a free-throw and warned the offending player.			
Learner signature:	Stephen Patrick	**Date:**	11\09\2012
Assessor signature:	Ann Coates	**Date:**	11\09\2012

Assessor report: The assessor has produced a detailed personalised observation statement which clearly demonstrates how the learner has applied the rules of handball in four situations. They have presented a clear description of the situation and how the learner responded in each situation.

Assessor report – overall

Is the evidence sufficient to satisfy the grading criterion?

The learner has presented evidence to show that they have been able to apply the rules of a sport in four specific situations. However, the observation statement needs to be backed up by video evidence so that the assessor can check that the grading criteria have been accurately applied.

What additional evidence, if any, is required?

To achieve 2A.P2 the assessor would need to check the video evidence against the witness statement.

Describe the roles and responsibilities of officials from two selected sports

✍ **Learner answer**

Handball

In handball there are two referees and they either take the role of field referee or goal referee. These referees are supported by a third referee, whose role is to record goals, track any suspensions and start and stop the clock.

The referees position themselves so that all the players are contained between them. They position themselves on opposite sides of the court so that each referee can observe one sideline. One referee is called the 'goal referee' and they will stand on the goal line at the end of the court being attacked. The other referee is called the 'field referee' and they position themselves on the court. They will change their role depending on which team is attacking. Their responsibilities are to start and restart play, indicate any infractions and apply necessary sanctions; they also decide if the ball crosses the line for a goal.

Badminton

In badminton there are six officials. There is one umpire who is in charge of the game and ensures the rules are applied correctly. They will also keep a record of the score. There are four line judges who make judgements about whether the shuttlecock is in play or not. There is also a service judge who ensures that the service is valid and at the correct height. All the officials will use hand signals to indicate the decision that they have made.

There can also be a match referee who manages the tournament and makes sure that the tournament is played fairly.

Assessor report – overall

What is good about this assessment evidence?

The candidate has chosen two sports and has described some of the
roles and responsibilities of officials for these sports.

What could be improved about this assessment evidence?

When discussing handball, the candidate could have outlined more
of the responsibilities of the referee and discussed the hand signals
that they use to indicate why they have made a decision. Also, there
are inaccuracies about the role of a 'third referee', as these roles are
taken by a scorekeeper and a time-keeper rather than a third referee.
These inaccuracies would need to be corrected to achieve P3. Again,
the badminton answer would have benefited from a more detailed
description of the responsibilities of the umpire.

2A.M1 For each of the two selected sports, explain the roles and responsibilities of officials and the application of rules, regulations and scoring systems

Assessor report: The command verb in the grading criterion is explain. In their answer we would expect to see that they had developed the points that they made for pass criteria and given more depth about the rules, regulations and scoring systems and the roles and responsibilities of officials. The criterion asks for application of the rules so we would expect to see examples of rules in action and the sanctions for breaking the rules.

✍ Learner answer

In handball the referees have to have a detailed knowledge of the rules and regulations and be able to apply them on the court of play. They are responsible for the behaviour of the players on the court and if they observe foul play or an infringement of the rules, they are able to apply sanctions such as a free-throw, a seven-metre throw or progressive punishments such as warnings (yellow card) or exclusion (red card). A free-throw is awarded if a team uses passive play, which is when a team keeps the ball without making any attempt to attack; this results in a free-throw to the opposition. Free-throws are awarded for minor fouls or minor rule violations. A 7-metre throw is a penalty throw and is awarded when a foul deprives a player of a clear chance to score, when a defensive player enters their own goal area or if the goalkeeper takes the ball into their goal area.

If a foul merits more action than just a free-throw, for example, if a player pushes another player to the ground, the referee can give a warning. If a player receives more than two warnings or a team receives more than three, any further warnings will result in the player being suspended for five minutes. An exclusion is given for repeated fouling or assault on another player and means the player must leave the game. They can be replaced on the court by another player after two minutes **(a)**.

The referees must also safeguard the health and safety of the players by ensuring that they have the correct clothing and equipment. Players are not allowed to wear jewellery or watches as they could be used to cause harm or injury to their opponent when their opponent comes in contact with their arms. Clothing is protective as well as being used to recognise the players on each team **(b)**. They will have to deal with any injuries that players sustain by stopping play and then allowing them to have the treatment they need. They are also responsible for communicating with the players. They do this by using a whistle to stop and start play, hand signals to indicate what they have awarded and their voice to explain any further information that is needed. This information is important to keep the game flowing and protect the safety of the players.

In badminton the umpire is in charge of the match and must enforce the rules of badminton. The umpire calls out any faults that the line or service judges indicate and they can overrule the line judges if they think they are wrong. The umpire tells the players and the audience the score after each point. They can stop play for an injury to allow for medical treatment. They also ensure the players behave themselves on court and can record any examples of misconduct and report them to the referee.

Assessor report – overall

What is good about this assessment evidence?

This is a good, detailed answer where the explanation of the roles and responsibilities of the officials are combined with the application of rules and regulations. The candidate gives examples of when the officials can apply sanctions – the example of a player pushing an opponent to the ground **(a)**. The sanctions that can be applied are clearly explained. The reasons behind the responsibilities of officials to check clothing and communication with the players are well explained **(b)**.

The roles and responsibilities of the umpire are well explained, with more information than was given for the pass criterion.

What could be improved about this assessment evidence?

When discussing handball, the candidate has included some inaccuracies in the information given about the number of warnings that result in a suspension, and the length of that suspension. The candidate would need to ensure that all of this information is correct to achieve M1.

The answer could have been improved by explaining the roles and responsibilities of the line judges and the match referee. Also there is only limited information about the application of the rules, with no examples given.

2A.D1 **Compare and contrast the roles and responsibilities of officials from two selected sports, suggesting valid recommendations for improvements to the application of rules, regulations and scoring systems for each sport**

Assessor report: The command verbs in the grading criterion are compare and contrast. In their answer we would expect a candidate to show what the similarities and what the differences are between the roles and responsibilities of the players.

Learner answer

Despite having different names (umpire and referee), the roles of both officials have many things in common. Firstly they both have to implement the rules of the sports and make judgements based on the rules. Secondly, they are both responsible for the health and safety of the players by checking their clothing, equipment and playing surfaces. Thirdly, both sets of officials have to communicate with their fellow officials by using hand signals and communicate with the players when necessary. Fourthly, the officials in both sports keep moving.

There are many differences as well between their roles and responsibilities. The handball referees change the role that they play depending on the position of play, while the badminton officials always do the same role. The umpire in badminton keeps the score and has assistants to help apply the rules; in handball the two referees are responsible for applying the rules but they have assistants to keep score and keep time. In handball the referees have total authority and can apply serious sanctions (warnings and expulsions) for misconduct; in badminton there is a higher authority than the umpire, the match referee, and the umpire has to report bad behaviour to the match referee.

The application of rules and regulations can be difficult in fast-moving sports such as handball and badminton. Badminton has six officials on the court and they are needed as the shuttlecock is small and moves very fast. In contrast, the two officials in handball have to watch 14 players on court, who may all be moving at the same time, and the ball, which may not be easy to see. They also have to keep moving and changing roles so they may benefit from having an extra official who stands on the side and watches the match. They may be able to help the court officials to make difficult decisions. The badminton umpire would benefit from another official keeping the score so that they can concentrate on ensuring that the rules of badminton are not broken. In tennis and cricket they use technology called 'Hawkeye' which is able to say where the ball has landed and it helps the officials with their line calls and decision making. This would help badminton officials decide whether the shuttlecock was in or out.

In badminton the scoring system has been changed. It used to be that the first player to 15 points was the winner and you could only score points when you served. This has been changed so that you can score on every point. It helps to make the game more attacking as a player wants to win every point rather than playing in a defensive way. In badminton the scoring system when both players reach 20 points could be changed. It is unfair that if the score is 29–29 then the next point wins. Badminton could have a tie-break system like tennis so when scores are tied at 21–21 they could play another 7 points to see who wins the game.

Assessor report – overall

What is good about this assessment evidence?

The candidate has clearly compared and contrasted the roles and responsibilities of the badminton and handball officials. The candidate also makes valid suggestions on how the officiating of the two sports could be improved by using other officials and technology. They also give some interesting ideas about how the scoring system in badminton could be further improved and explained how and why it has been changed in the past.

What could be improved about this assessment evidence?

The candidate has included more similarities than differences in the officials' roles and responsibilities, and suggesting that officials in both sports keep moving is incorrect. They need to correct these details and show an equal number of similarities and differences. There is no reference to the scoring system in handball and even if the student does not feel it needs to be changed at all, they need to say this and explain why.

Learning aim B

Practically demonstrate skills, techniques and tactics in selected sports

Assessment criteria

2B.P4   Describe the technical and tactical demands of two selected sports.

2B.P5   Use relevant skills and tactics effectively, in two selected sports, in conditioned practices.

2A.M2   Use relevant skills, techniques and tactics effectively, in competitive situations.

Topic B.1 Technical demands

The technical demands of a sport are the different skills/techniques that are needed to be effective in playing a sport. For example, in badminton a player needs to be able to serve, play lob shots, drop shots and smashes.

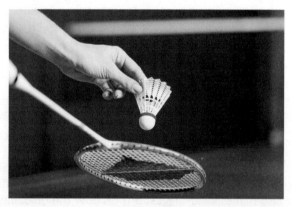

Figure 5.1

Continuous skills

Studied ☐

Continuous skills are those that have no clear beginning or end as the end of one skill leads into the start of the next. They tend to be rhythmical in nature such as running, skipping, cycling, rowing or using a step machine.

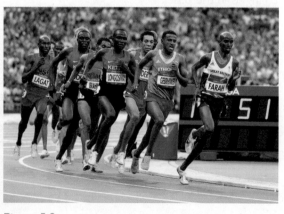

Figure 5.2

Discrete skills

Studied ☐

Discrete skills are those skills with a clear beginning and end. They are performed in a single effort such as a basketball free throw, tennis serve or a shot in cricket.

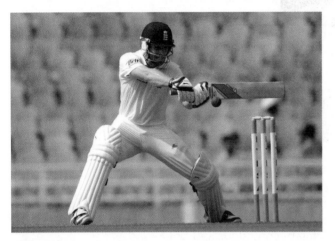

Figure 5.3

Serial skills

Studied ☐

Serial skills consist of a number of discrete or continuous skills put together. For example, a triple jump combines a run up, hop, skip, jump and landing. Other examples include a dribble and shoot in basketball or a synchronised swimming routine.

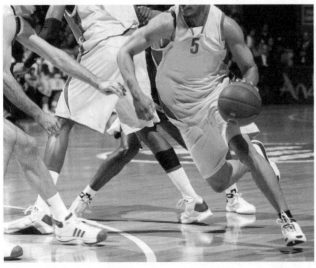

Figure 5.4

Topic B.2 Tactical demands

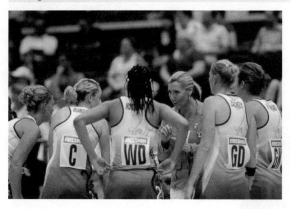

Figure 5.5

Tactics are the plans that you put in place and execute to increase your chances of winning. They can relate to decision making, methods of defending and attacking, the choice of shots or strokes you make, how you vary your play in different conditions and how you use space, and any other demands that are specific to your sport.

Topic B.3 Safe and appropriate participation

Skills, techniques and tactics need to be demonstrated in a safe and appropriate environment. This means that checks have been made to ensure that the facilities are safe, the equipment is safe and well maintained and that the participants are free from injury and healthy. The environment will be controlled, meaning that the session will be non-competitive and include drills and set plays.

Topic B.4 Relevant skills and techniques

The skills and techniques that are used to perform a sport and practices for that sport will be demonstrated practically. For example, if tennis was your chosen sport, you would need to be able to show that you can serve, play forehands and backhands, lobs and drop shots. You should be able to play both ground strokes and volleys.

Topic B.5 Relevant tactics

The tactics that are used to perform in a sport also need to be demonstrated. For example, in tennis you could demonstrate different serves and volleys, and tactics for defensive and attacking play.

Topic B.6 Effective use of skills and techniques, and the correct application of each component

You need to be able to demonstrate that you can use skills and techniques for your chosen sport effectively, and that you can apply them correctly. For example, in a tennis serve you could show correct body position, the ball toss, the backswing, connecting with the ball, follow through and moving into position to receive the return.

Topic B.7 Effective use of skills, techniques and tactics

You need to show the effective use of skills and techniques within conditioned (non-competitive) and competitive situations, showing effective decision making and appropriate selection of skills, techniques and tactics when being placed under pressure by your opponent.

Topic B.8 Isolated practices

Isolated practice is when you take a skill and practise it outside a game situation. For example, a cricketer practising in the nets or a badminton player practising serves without an opponent. Isolated practices are used to focus on specific skills within a sport and then the performer needs to transfer these skills into competitive situations.

Topic B.9 Conditioned practices

Conditioned practices are when a sport is changed to focus practice on certain skills/techniques. For example, playing small-sided games to focus on one touch passing or practising tennis only using backhand shots.

Topic B.10 Competitive situations

Competitive situations are when the sport is played is its full form with an opposition and match officials.

Knowledge recap

1. Describe the technical demands of a sport.
2. Describe the difference between continuous and discrete skills.
3. Describe the difference between conditioned practice and competitive situations.

Assessment guidance for learning aim B

Scenario

As part of your work with the summer sports scheme you need to prepare a hand-out for the children that describes the techniques and tactics of the two sports that you are going to play. Before playing these sports you will need to show your manager that you can demonstrate the techniques and tactics.

2B.P4 **Describe the technical and tactical demands of two selected sports**

Assessor report: The command verb in the grading criterion is **describe**. In the answer we would expect to see a detailed account of the technical and tactical demands of a team and an individual sport.

 Learner answer

Handball

Technical demands

To play handball well a player has to be able to do the following:

- Catch the ball at different heights.
- Pass over short and long distances.
- Move quickly around the court.
- Change direction quickly.
- Catch and pass the ball while running.
- Shoot from different positions.
- Free themselves from their defender.
- Work as part of the team.
- Dribble with the ball.

Tactical demands

In handball the tactical demands relate to how the team defends and attacks. Some teams defend using man-to-man defence where each player has an opponent to defend against.

Zone defence means that a player has a certain space to defend and they defend when an opponent comes into their zone. Combined defence is used when the opposition have a star player and five players use zone defence and one player uses man-to-man marking on the star player. Attacking tactics include fast attack when the team have to get a player into a shooting position as fast as they can. The goal keeper will play a fast throw to the left or right and they will play a fast ball to the shooter before the defenders can get back.

Badminton

In badminton the techniques are:

- serve
- clears
- drop shots
- smash
- drive
- net play.

The tactics are different between singles and doubles but the main thing is to get your opponent moving around the court in different ways. This is very good if they are not mobile or not very fit.

The first one is movement pressure which is created by moving your opponent around in different ways:

- Hitting to the corners, which is moving the player from the central base to the four corners.
- Use long diagonals, which means moving your player from the backhand front court to the forehand rear court.
- Force your opponent to change direction from forwards to backwards or from side to side.

Assessor report: The work on handball is good and the technical and tactical demands are well described, but the work on badminton is not detailed enough. Stating the techniques does not meet the criterion to 'describe' and you would need to add in some extra information to describe the techniques, providing a similar level of detail as is given for handball. For example, you could say that a drop shot is one that falls into the frontcourt to bring your opponent to the front of the court so that you can then hit towards the back of the court; or serves can be high serves, low serves, backhand and flick serves. The tactics are good but you could add in tactics for other techniques, such as serving.

2B.P5 Use relevant skills and tactics effectively, in two selected sports, in conditioned practices

2A.M2 Use relevant skills, techniques and tactics effectively, in competitive situations

Assessor report: For these two assessment criteria the assessment is done in practical situations. You will have to show that you can use techniques and tactics in real, practical situations. You can gather your evidence in a range of ways within your school/college.

Firstly, your teacher can watch you performing in two sports of your choice and then complete a witness observation sheet. You may also use video or photographic evidence to demonstrate your participation in a sport and using techniques and tactics.

If you are not able to demonstrate all the techniques and tactics, you can use a log book that you fill in to describe when and how you have used them. You could use photographs in your log book to show you using a particular technique or tactic.

Your teacher may allow you to gather evidence when you play for your club through videos of your performances backed up by witness statements from your coach where they describe what they saw you doing during play. You can also use a commentary to describe what you were doing and show how you have met the assessment criteria.

It is important to note that to achieve a Merit you will need to demonstrate your use of techniques and tactics in a full, competitive situation. To achieve a Pass you can demonstrate your skills in a practice situation. Also to achieve the assessment criteria you need to be observed in two selected sports.

Learning aim C
Be able to review sports performance

Assessment criteria

2C.P6	Independently produce an observation checklist that can be used effectively to review own performance in two selected sports.
2C.P7	Review own performance in two selected sports, describing strengths and areas for improvement.
2C.M3	Explain strengths and areas for improvement in two selected sports, recommending activities to improve own performance.
2C.D2	Analyse strengths and areas of improvement in two selected sports, justifying recommended activities to improve own performance.

Topic C.1 Observation checklist

An observation checklist is a document that is prepared by a coach or performer to enable them to record as much information as they can about an individual or a team's performance.

It can be used by a performer to self-analyse their performance and then to identify areas of strength and areas for improvement.

It can be used to observe behaviour when watching a sports performance live or by a video recording. A video recording enables the coach or performer to watch and re-watch the performance so that they can gain as much information as is possible.

The observation checklist can be used to observe:

- Technical demands of a sport – for example, number of passes, shots, tackles, headers and blocks. The checklist should include information about whether the technique was performed successfully or unsuccessfully and also the different types of each technique, such as defensive or attacking headers, long or short passes.
- Tactical demands of a sport – this would focus on the decision making, choice of shots or strokes, positional requirements of the sport and tactics specific to the team or individual situation.

Topic C.2 Review performance

Reviewing performance is important so you can identify what you do well (areas of strength) and what you could improve on and to pick out specific aspects of your play that you need to work on (areas for improvement). A good review will consider your sport-specific skills and techniques, tactics, fitness and psychological skills.

Information about your performance can look at the outcome of your play, such as the number of goals that you have scored or the number of first serves that were successful. Also you need to look at the process of your play, that is how well you performed the skills and how they felt to perform. It is very useful to get feedback from other people, such as your coach, team mates and other observers.

Once you have reviewed your performance and found out your areas of strength and areas for improvement, you can set yourself short-term and long-term goals aimed at tackling any areas for improvement. These goals need to be supported by activities to increase performance in the areas for improvement. These activities can be included in your training programme along with other activities such as attending training or coaching courses, seeking specialist advice from experts or using technology to help you improve.

Knowledge recap

1. Why is it important to review your own performance?

2. Where can you gain information about your performance?

Assessment guidance for learning aim C

Scenario

During your work at the summer holiday sports scheme you will need to develop the children's techniques and tactics. In order to do this effectively, you need to be able to show that you can develop your own techniques and tactics.

2C.P6 **Independently produce an observation checklist that can be used effectively to review own performance in two selected sports**

Assessor report: The command verb here is **independently produce**. This means that you need to design an observation checklist without the support of your teacher.

 Learner answer

Observation checklist for handball

Technique	Tally	Score out of 10	Comment
Successful passes			
Unsuccessful passes			
Shots on target			
Shots off target			
Goals			
Tackles made			
Tackles missed			
Interceptions			
Entries into attacking zone			
Mistakes leading to goals			
Fouls			
Penalties conceded			

Observation checklist for badminton

Technique	Tally	Score out of 10	Comment
Smash			
Overhead clear			
Forehand shots			
Backhand shots			
Net shots			
Tactics			
Offensive play			
Defensive play			
Hitting corners			
Getting opponent to change direction			

Assessor report: These are basic checklists and cover the main features of the sports you will review. There are many more techniques in badminton than have been covered, such as shots from the back of the court. You could have added in some tactics to your checklist for handball. It would also have been worthwhile to add in some psychological aspects such as decision making (shot selection) and controlling anxiety/nerves.

Review own performance in two selected sports, describing strengths and areas for improvement

✎ **Learner answer**

Performance review for handball

Technique	Tally	Score out of 10	Comment
Successful passes	||||||||||||||||||||	8	Pleased with my passing – most passes were successful
Unsuccessful passes	||||		
Shots on target	||||||||||	7	
Shots off target	|||||		
Goals	|||	5	Should be scoring more goals with the number of shots I had
Tackles made	||||||||||||	6	
Tackles missed	||||||		Need to make more tackles
Interceptions	||||||||||	8	Very pleased with this
Entries into attacking zone	||||||||||||||||||||	7	Getting into good attacking positions
Mistakes leading to goals	||||	3	This is not acceptable
Fouls	||||||||	3	Too many fouls conceded
Penalties conceded			3	If I had not made a mistake I would not have needed to give away a penalty

My strength is my passing as I was successful with most of my passes and I got most of my shots on target. I need to keep working on my shooting as I am not scoring enough goals for the number of shots I have. I am getting into good positions in the attacking zone and that is why I am having a lot of shots.

My area that needs improvement is my defensive work.

In summary I need to work more on thinking about the defensive side of my game and preventing goals rather than always trying to get into goal-scoring positions. I need to play more for the team rather than for my own glory.

Learning aim C: Be able to review sports performance

Performance review for Badminton

Technique	Successful	Unsuccessful	Comment
Smash	IIIIIIIIIIIIIII	III	I am really confident when I play smashes
Overhead clear	IIIIII	IIIIIIIIIII	I keep thinking too much about overhead shots and then mess them up
Drop shots	IIIIII	IIIIIIIIII	Too many of my drop shots go wide
Forehand shots	IIIIIIIIIIIIIIIIIIIIIIIIIII IIII	III	I love playing shots on my forehand and avoid backhands if I can
Backhand shots	IIIIIIIII	IIIIIIIII	I keep making mistakes with my backhand shots
Net shots	IIIIIIIIIIIIIII	IIIII	

Tactics	Score /10	Strengths	Weaknesses
Offensive play	8	Attacking the net and using smashes	
Defensive play	4		I get bored playing defensive shots and keep wanting to attack my opponent
Hitting corners	6	I am good at hitting the back corners, particularly the right hand corner	I am not so good at hitting the front corners with drop shots and often hit the shuttle too hard
Getting opponent to change direction	3		I concentrate too much on playing to my strengths rather than thinking what my opponent is doing

My strengths are my attacking game and playing smashes from the front of the court; I am very good at turning defensive play into attacking play and putting pressure on my opponent to make mistakes.

My weakness is that I avoid playing certain shots that I am not very good at, such as backhand shots. I need to think more about making it difficult for my opponent by moving them around the court more and getting them to make mistakes that way.

Assessor report – overall

What is good about this assessment evidence?

These checklists have been clearly filled in and identify and describe areas where the candidate feels strong and areas that need improving.

What could be improved about this assessment evidence?

The answers are slightly limited because the checklists are short on detail. For handball, the candidate has stated that their defensive work needs improvement, but has not gone on to **describe** this area for improvement. They could, for example, have explained that because they want to get into attacking situations, they make mistakes in defence, and have to commit fouls to make up for bad positioning. They would need to fully describe this area for improvement in order to achieve P7.

Explain strengths and areas for improvement in two selected sports, recommending activities to improve own performance

Assessor report: The command verb here is **explain**. This means that you need to give a detailed account of your areas of strength and those that need improving. You would also need to explain why they are a strength/area for improvement and give examples of how improvement could be made.

 Learner answer

Handball

My main strength is my passing and I know this because I have many more successful passes than unsuccessful ones. My passing is always at the right height and right speed for my teammate to catch without slowing down **(a)**. Also, my shots on target are a strength and when I have a shot, my checklist shows that I normally get it on target **(a)**. Shooting is a weakness as well as I don't score as many goals as I should do **(b)**. I need to practise shooting at different parts of the goal and from different positions. I also need to learn how to feint and make the goalkeeper think I am going to do one thing and actually do another **(c)**.

I am very good at making interceptions and I made 9 out of the 10 that I tried. This is because I am tall and have long arms to intercept the ball **(a)**.

My main area of weakness is my defence and we use zone defence. I am not very good at staying in my zone and get excited when the ball moves forwards. I always move to the ball and join in with the attack, leaving my zone empty for the opposition to attack **(b)**.

Badminton

My main strengths are in my attacking shots and then shots I use to win a point. In particular I am very confident in playing smashes and nearly always win a point, except when I hit it too hard and it goes out. My forehand shots are very accurate and always go the part of the court that I want them to. I am good at forehands because I like to practise them **(a)**.

Backhand shots are my weakness as I don't get enough power in them and am not good at directing them **(b)**. I need to have some practice sessions where a coach makes me only play backhands and keeps hitting onto my backhand **(c)**. My drop shots are an area that needs improving because I keep hitting them too hard and they go out of play at the side.

My overhead clears were too hard as well and I was unsuccessful with a lot of them – they are used to push the player to the back of the court but I often hit them too hard and put them out past the back line **(b)**.

I need to relax more on court and not be so aggressive with my shots and hit them too hard **(c)**.

Assessor report – overall

What is good about this assessment evidence?

There is a very good explanation of the candidate's strengths for both selected sports **(a)**. There is also a particularly good explanation of areas that need improvement **(b)**. Some good examples of practice that could be undertaken in order to work on the areas that need improvement are also provided **(c)**.

What could be improved about this assessment evidence?

The candidate has not explained what activities they could complete to improve their performance in defence when playing handball. They could have suggested some drills here that would help them when deciding when to go forward and when to stay in defence. In order to achieve M3, the candidate needs to include recommendations for activities to improve performance for all areas needing improvement.

2C.D2 Analyse strengths and areas of improvement in two selected sports, justifying recommended activities to improve own performance

Assessor report: The command verb here is **analyse**. This means that you need to look at the reasons why something is a strength or an area for improvement. In this question you need to give examples of practices that will address these areas for improvement and explain why they would be effective.

 Learner answer

Handball

My passing is my main strength because I always get the speed and accuracy right and pick the right pass. My teammate is always able to catch the ball without having to stop or slow down. I don't need to practise passes so much **(a)**.

My shooting is an area that needs improving, although it looks like a strength, as I have good accuracy and get the shot on target, but I don't get enough goals. This is because I don't think about placing the shot as I aim to get power and to get them on target **(b)**. For these reasons I will organise some practice where I put targets in the top and bottom corners and aim to hit them from different shooting positions. This will help me to vary my shots and direct them away from the goalkeeper into the corners **(c)**.

My defending is poor because I am to blame for too many goals and fouls as I get out of position because I like to attack **(b)**. I need to practise defending as part of the team and learn the tactics and in what situations I should go and attack and in what situations I can defend. Then I need to practise these in game situations. Then I will become better at defending and the team will lose fewer goals **(c)**.

Badminton

My main strengths are my smashes as I always pick the right time to play them and hardly ever hit them into the net. I win lots of points with smashes and like hitting the shuttle hard. Sometime I hit them too hard and they go out; then I know I have to calm down a bit. My forehand shots are a strength as well as

I am powerful and accurate with them and hit them to the right part of the court.

My backhands are my area for improvement. I know because I only play them when I have to and if I can move to play a backhand on a forehand then I do.

Assessor report – overall

What is good about this assessment evidence?

There is some very good work here. The work on handball clearly analyses why the candidate's strengths are strengths by explaining what it is about the passes that make them strengths and the effect this has on teammates – that they can catch the ball and not stop or slow down **(a)**. For areas of improvement the candidate explains why they are weak **(b)** and also gives some excellent practice sessions that will help you to improve in these areas, justifying why they will help to improve performance **(c)**.

What could be improved about this assessment evidence?

The work on badminton is not as good as the work on handball and does not improve on the work completed for the merit criteria. The candidate has not thought about why the backhands are a weakness – what they are doing badly and what the outcome is of the backhands. Then they need to explain practice sessions that could be done to improve the backhands. Also, they need to analyse their drop shots and overhead clears and what it is that they do badly in these shots and practices and what they could do to improve these techniques. They would need to provide this missing detail for badminton in order to achieve D2.

Sample assignment brief

PROGRAMME NAME:		BTEC First Certificate/Extended Certificate in Sport UNIT 2: Practical Sports Performance
TUTOR NAME:		
STUDENT NAME:		
DATE SET:		SUBMISSION DATE:

This assignment will assess the following learning aims:

A Understand the rules, regulations and scoring systems for selected sports.

B Practically demonstrate skills, techniques and tactics in sport.

C Be able to review sports performance.

Scenario

You want to secure a holiday job working as a coach at a sports camp for 8–13 year olds. As part of this process, you need to be able to show to your potential employer that you have both knowledge of selected sports and expertise in performing and officiating selected sports. You have been asked to complete a series of tasks to demonstrate your skills and knowledge of two sports.

Task 1

a) Present a handbook that describes the roles and responsibilities of officials in two sports and describe the rules, regulations and scoring systems in the two selected sports. You need to explain the roles and responsibilities of officials and the application of rules, regulations and scoring systems. You need to compare and contrast the roles of responsibilities from two selected sports and make valid recommendations for the improvement of the application of rules, regulations and scoring system for each sport.

b) Present observation records, witness statements or video evidence to show that you have been able to apply the rules in a selected sport in four different situations.

Task 2

a) Produce an A3-sized poster describing the technical and tactical demands of two selected sports.

b) Present observation records, witness statements or video evidence to demonstrate that you are able to use effectively relevant skills, techniques and tactics in two selected sports in conditioned practice. You need to demonstrate these relevant skills, techniques and tactics in two selected sports in competitive situations.

Task 3

a) Using your knowledge of effective performance in two sports, produce independently a checklist that can be used to review your own performance in each sport.

b) Having designed two checklists that can be used to effectively review performance in different sports, use the checklists to review your performance and describe your strengths and areas for improvements in each selected sport. You need to explain your strengths and areas for improvement in your two selected sports and recommend activities that you can do to improve your own performance. You need to analyse your strengths and areas for improvement in your two selected sports and justify the activities you have recommended to improve your own performance.

Assessment criteria

Level 2 Pass	Level 2 Merit	Level 3 Distinction
Learning aim A: Understand the rules, regulations and scoring systems for selected sports.		
2A.P1 Describe the rules, regulations and scoring systems of two selected sports.	**2A.M1** For each of the two selected sports, explain the role and responsibilities of officials and the application of rules, roles and scoring systems.	**2A.D1** Compare and contrast the roles and responsibilities of officials from two selected sports, suggesting valid recommendations for improvement to the rules, regulations and scoring systems for each sport.
2A.P2 Apply the rules of a selected sport in four specific situations.		
2A.P3 Describe the roles and responsibilities of officials from two selected sports.		
Learning aim B: Practically demonstrate skills, techniques and tactics in selected sports.		
2B.P4 Describe the technical and tactical demands of two selected sports.		
2B.P5 Use relevant skills, techniques and tactics effectively, in two selected sports, in conditioned practices.	**2B.M2** Use relevant skills, techniques and tactics effectively, in two selected sports, in competitive practices.	
Learning aim C: Be able to review sports performance.		
2C.P6 Independently produce an observation checklist that can be used effectively to review own performance in two selected sports.		
2D.P7 Review own performance in two selected sports, identifying strengths and areas for improvement.	**2D.M3** Explain strengths and areas for improvement in two selected sports, recommending activities to improve own performance.	**2D.D2** Analyse strengths and areas for improvement in two selected sports, justifying recommended activities to improve own performance.

Unit 1 External assessment: Answers for question paper 1

1. **(b)** specificity

2. **(b)** circuit training

3. **(b)** speed.

4. Flexibility

5. Progression; Adaptation; Reversibility; Variation; Rest.

6. **(a)** continuous training.
   (b) interval training.

7. **(a)** Target zone is the level of intensity that must be reached during training to make exercise worthwhile.
   (b) It is calculated from 220 minus your age **(1)**, then you would exercise at a level between 60% and 80% of this figure **(1)**.

8. **(a)** Wear the correct clothing and footwear **(1)**. Make sure that the activity area is safe, no water on the floor, no rubbish or kit left in the way **(1)**.
   (b) Wearing the correct clothing and footwear: when using equipment in the gym you must wear trainers and sports clothing so that you do not trip or catch your clothing on machines **(1)**. You must make sure that the activity playing area is free from obstacles so that no one slips or trips and falls, causing an injury **(1)**.

9. **(d)** Aerobic fitness.

10. The role of the cardiorespiratory system is to take in oxygen from the air we breathe **(1)**, to transport nutrients and oxygen around the body **(1)** and to remove waste products including carbon dioxide **(1)**.

11. As training progresses, our body adapts to the new level of fitness. If we do not continue to push our bodies and work them harder we will not progress. For fitness levels to increase, the body must work harder, the training programme must be adapted to ensure progress. A netball player might be using an aerobic training programme to help her to develop her aerobic fitness. If she has a higher level of aerobic fitness, she will be able to run and perform at a higher level for longer. After six weeks the netballer will see that she has progressed, she has become fitter and can complete her aerobic training easily. It is important that she increases her aerobic training so that she continues to improve and increase her fitness. If the netballer had been training three times a week and training for one hour, she could now train for longer and more times a week. She could also increase the intensity that she works at, for example, if she uses the treadmill and runs at level 6, she could increase this to level 7.

12. **(a)** the vertical jump test
    (b) power
    (c) hand grip test or hand grip dynamometer
    (d) strength.

13. **(a)** Strength training exercises should be followed by stretching because as the muscles work they tear **(1)**; tearing causes the muscles to rebuild and grow **(1)**; if the muscles are not stretched during training they will re-grow closer together and the muscles will become shorter **(1)**.
    (b) The sit and reach test **(1)** requires a person to sit with legs straight in front of them touching a sit and reach box **(1)**, the person has to reach as far forward as they can, keeping their legs straight **(1)**; the distance reached on the sit and reach box is recorded; this is usually repeated and an average of the results is recorded **(1)**.

14. **(a)** A weight training programme designed to build up strength will involve using heavy weights **(1)** and performing a small number of repetitions **(1)**.
    (b) Rugby; Boxing; Weight lifting; Discus throwing.

15. Rugby; Netball; Tennis; Swimming.

16. When carrying out a fitness test the same instructions should be used **(1)**; the test should use the same equipment **(1)**, which has been standardised for the test **(1)**; the testing environment should be the same when the test is repeated, e.g. if the bleep test is carried out on the sports field it should be re-tested there **(1)**.

17. **(a)** body fat callipers.
    (b) measuring body fat percentage.

18. **(a)** cm or inches
    (b) average.

Markscheme for 8-mark questions

Level	Mark	Descriptor
0	0	No rewardable material
1	1–3	Answers will include a basic description of how training can be increased to ensure progression. Limited understanding of how the body systems will change and adapt to an increasing level of exercise.
2	4–6	Answers will include a sound explanation of how training can be increased to ensure progression. There will be a good level of understanding which demonstrates good knowledge of the body systems and the importance of progressing a training programme to ensure the body becomes fitter.
3	7–8	Answers will include a detailed discussion of how training can be increased to ensure progression. There will be a detailed discussion which demonstrates a very good knowledge of the body systems and the importance of progressing a training programme to ensure the body becomes fitter. Relevant sport specific examples will be included throughout the answer.

Unit 1 External assessment: Answers for question paper 2

1. **(d)** type.

2. Reaction time is the time taken for a performer to react to a stimulus and initiate a response. Being fast off the blocks is important as the race is short. Faster reaction time means faster performance.

3. Advantages – large groups tested at once, quick and easy to perform. Disadvantages – having feet held can affect validity as increases role of hip flexors and does not measure ab strength, sometimes difficult to see if the correct sit-up is performed and there may be dispute about the total number.

4. **(a) (i)** resistance
   (b) (iii) muscular endurance.

5. AGILITY – The ability of a sports performer to move quickly and precisely or change direction without losing balance or time.
   POWER – The product of strength and speed.

6. **(a)** Providing different activities within the training plan.
   (b) To prevent boredom and maintain enjoyment.

7. **(a)** $220 - 18 \times 0.6 = 121$ and $220 - 18 \times 0.85 = 172$
   (b) RPE is a rating of how hard you feel your body is working. An approximation of heart rate on this scale would be to multiply the effort level by 10. This would put the RPE value at the upper limit at 17.

8. **(b)** squat, seated row, calf raise, bicep curl.

9. REPETITION – is one performance of a single exercise.
   SETS – comprise a number of exercise repetitions performed without stopping.

10. **(d)** plyometrics.

11. **(a)** sit and reach
    (b) flexibility
    (c) validity – the sit and reach only measures the flexibility of the lower back and hamstrings and therefore it cannot be used to assess the flexibility of other areas of the body.
    Reliability – the range of movement is affected by the extent of the warm-up. If properly warmed up, the scores will be higher than if there is no warm-up provided.

12. BMI; bioelectrical impedence; skinfold testing.

13. Boys – chest, abdomen and thigh.
    Girls – triceps, suprailiac and thigh.

14. Award up to eight marks for describing the following factors. Personal information including age, ability, lifestyle factors, current fitness levels and activity. Personal training goals and targets need to be established. Inclusion and consideration of FITT principles. Specific training methods to be considered such as resistance training relevant to the specific activity. Timescales and the availability of resources. Session content including warm-up, cool-down, technique. Additional principles of training to include overload, adaptation, rest, reversibility. Variation in planning and in activities to prevent boredom.

15. **(a)** 49.3
    (b) see norm table used
    (c) (i) ml/kg/min.

16. circuit training.

17.

Exercise	1 RM	Reps	Sets	Weight
Squat	150 kg	6	3	135 kg

18. Fitness testing provides a baseline for monitoring improvement and performance levels as any future testing could be compared to the original score to establish progress. Fitness testing can help in the design of programmes because they can establish the training needs of athletes so that training can be planned to address the areas for improvement. They can also be used to see if programmes are working by identifying if there are changes in the fitness scores. Fitness testing can be used to set goals by providing quantifiable markers for improvement so that the athlete can work towards those goals.

Unit 2 Knowledge recap answers

Learning aim A, page 71

1. Rules are an agreed set of standards laid down to standardise how a sport is played.
2. A governing body will decide on the rules of a sport and appoint officials to implement the rules.
3. Tennis umpires will i) call the score; ii) rule whether a ball is in or out of play and iii) call any 'let' serves.

Learning aim B, page 87

1. The technical demands are the different skills/techniques that are needed to perform the sport effectively.
2. A discrete skill is one with a clear start and finish while in a continuous skill, the end of one skill becomes the beginning of the next.

3. Conditioned practice occurs when a sport is modified to allow the player to focus on certain skills within the sport while a competitive situation involves the full game and uses all the skills/techniques of the sport.

Learning aim C, page 92

1. It is important to review your performance so that you can identify any areas for improvement that you need to work on.
2. You can gain information about your performance from your coach, teammates and any observers; you can also gain information by looking at the results of your play and how it felt to perform the skills/techniques.

Picture credits

The authors and publishers would like to thank the following for the use of photographs in this volume:

Figure 1.1 © Mikael Damkier – Fotolia; Figure 1.3 © Tyler Olson – Fotolia; Figure 1.4 © shotsstudio – Fotolia; Figure 1.5 © berc – Fotolia; Figure 1.7 © Ross Land/Getty Images; Figure 1.8 © Robi8 – Fotolia; Figure 1.9 © Friday – Fotolia; Figure 1.10 © Galina Barskaya – Fotolia; Figure 1.11 © Peter Kim – Fotolia; Figure 1.13 © Martinan – Fotolia; Figures in diagram on page 14 © Monkey Business – Fotolia (upper right), Ljupco Smokovski – Fotolia (bottom right), lassedesignen – Fotolia (bottom left), lilufoto – Fotolia (upper left); Figure 2.1 © Minerva Studio – Fotolia; Figure 2.2 © berc – Fotolia; Figure 2.9 © Dmitry Vereshchagin – Fotolia; Figure 2.10 © Elenathewise – Fotolia; Figure 2.11 © sumnersgraphicsinc – Fotolia; Figure 2.12 © Leo Mason/Corbis; Figure 2.13 © Getty Images/Stock4B Creative; Figure 3.6, also used on page 58, © Marcin / Sylwia C. / Fotolia. com; Figure 3.8 © Iconica/Getty Images; Figure 3.9 © CandyBox Images – Fotolia; Figure 3.10 © Ken Hurst – Fotolia; Figure 3.11 © alexandre zveiger – Fotolia; Figure on page 51 and page 66 © Novastock / Rex Features; Figure on page 56 © MARTYN F. CHILLMAID/ SCIENCE PHOTO LIBRARY; Figure on page 59 © Image Source IS2 – Fotolia; Figure 4.2 © Back Page Images / Rex Features; Figure 4.4 © Maxisport – Fotolia; Figure 5.1 © Kzenon – Fotolia; Figure 5.2 © KeystoneUSA-ZUMA / Rex Features; Figure 5.3 © INDRANIL MUKHERJEE/AFP/Getty Images; Figure 5.4 © Mariano Pozo Ruiz – Fotolia; Figure 5.5 © Daniel Swee / Alamy.

Every effort has been made to trace and acknowledge ownership of copyright. The publishers will be glad to make suitable arrangements with any copyright holders whom it has not been possible to contact.